mum, i wish i was dead

the story of a teenager who
conquered depression

ADAM SCHWARTZ

with Aniva Lee

D1388879

First published for Adam Schwartz by

Publish-*Me!*

A Division of
Longueville Media
PO Box 205
Haberfield NSW 2045 Australia
www.longmedia.com.au
info@longmedia.com.au
T. +61 2 9362 8441

National Library of Australia Cataloguing-in-Publication entry:

Creator:	Schwartz, Adam, author.
Title:	Mum, I wish I was dead : the story of a teenager who conquered depression / Adam Schwartz with Aviva Lowy.
ISBN:	9780994269102 (paperback)
Subjects:	Schwartz, Adam.
	Depression in adolescence--Australia--Biography.
	Depressed persons--Australia--Biography.
Other Creators/Contributors:	
	Lowy, Aviva, author.
Dewey Number:	616.852700835

To all those who have suffered and continue to suffer.
To all those who have cared and continue to care.

Acknowledgements

We all have a story to tell and despite this book revolving around my journey with depression, it is a story that could not have been told without help from others.

I thank my father Tony, mother Anne and brother Nathan for their unwavering support and love, both through my darkest times and every moment since: you loved me even when I wasn't very loveable. Thanks also to my grandparents who have played a significant role in my survival and growth as a person, and to my extended family and friends who have supported me and my family when we needed it most. To my new friends who never experienced my lowest points, I thank you for your love and support throughout sharing this story.

I thank Michael Visontay, who showed faith in me after our first meeting and for your continued support in producing and managing this entire project. Without you I wouldn't have had the pleasure of meeting Aviva Lowy, who took my story and captured the words I spoke to create a book that has such meaning. Without the both of you, my story would have remained unheard and all the potential help it can provide would have never been possible.

Thanks to my psychiatrist, Hugh Morgan, whose knowledge and support has been a constant point of hope and progress in my journey. To my clinical psychologist, Nick Cocco, you have played a huge role in my recovery and a significant part in maintaining my good health since.

Thanks are also needed for the doctors and nurses, both in and out of hospital and to my teachers, who helped me as much as they could during my school years. I apologise if there are people I have not specifically mentioned. However, to everyone who supported me at my lowest moments, I owe my survival to you. There will never be enough words to truly encapsulate my deepest thanks and appreciation for all that has been done.

Contents

1

Why I Wrote this Book

I have wanted to write this book for a very long time …

When I first recovered, I was so excited about being happy again that I wanted to share my insights and success with others. I did that through talking with friends, my personal training clients and parents who were concerned about their own kids.

The more I talked, the more people kept asking. As I spoke to doctors and other health professionals, I realised that I'd been particularly lucky. You see, the fact is I am a young male who has recovered from depression and is off medication.

Although rates of depression are higher in females than males, the suicide rate in males is significantly higher. Males are more likely to suppress their emotions. They have to toughen up or else get teased for expressing their feelings. And if your feelings are out of whack, then you are trapped trying to deal with them on your own.

Fortunately for me, I have always been comfortable about expressing how I feel and not being ashamed about being open with my emotions. It meant I was able to seek assistance and talk through my problems. Without a doubt, it allowed me to be open to the help that saved my life.

So expressing my emotions not only helped me to be one of those people who succeeds at beating depression, it meant that I could talk about the experience to others who are still stuck in the abyss. I've been there and I've done that. I am that guy who has jumped out of the aeroplane and I can tell you what it's like.

When I say 'beaten' depression, I mean that I can manage my depression using the many tools I have learned and developed so that depression no longer affects my day-to-day life.

Over the years I've always been open and happy to share my story. My mother would come to me and say, 'Someone has heard about you and they are worried about their child. Do you mind speaking to them?' I was always more than willing to do so.

The more people I spoke to, the more I realised how many people were suffering with depression even if they did not know it themselves. Suicide rates are unacceptably high. Every year in Australia more than 2500 people die through suicide and the numbers are not decreasing. This is a disease that modern medicine is unable to cure. Suicide is the number one killer of people aged 15 to 44.

According to the World Health Organisation, depression is the leading cause of disability worldwide. (The organisation claims that it was the second leading cause of death among 15–29 year olds globally in 2012.) Depression is the number one cause of non-fatal disability in Australia and one in seven Australians will suffer with depression in their lifetime.

To me, that's an epidemic. Why aren't elections being won based on what politicians plan to do to fix this problem? Is it because the public is unaware of the extent of this misery? Depression not only affects the individual, but it has a direct impact on the family, carers, friends, teachers and anyone coming into contact with them.

In the few short years since I struggled with depression, the resources available to help people have increased, including amazing online assistance that can be accessed for those living in remote areas or simply stuck at home. There are experts who can explain the science of what is happening to you and can give you tools to deal with it.

However, the gaps in the literature are the experiences of young people suffering and their battles and successes in overcoming this debilitating disease. Stories with sad outcomes tend to be highlighted and there are not enough positive experiences shared.

For almost any ailment, there are any number of people ready to share their story. They almost brag about their knee or shoulder surgeries and their success, or are comfortable to tell you what heart medications they are on and talk about their physical health. But they don't talk about their mental health. No one is rushing to let you know they've been depressed.

But if you are depressed, that's exactly the person you want to hear from. As vital as doctors are for the treatment of mental health, sometimes a person who has lived it can be a more comforting and reassuring voice.

A new mother who has just given birth may consult a large library written by parental experts on how to handle her baby, but she knows the best advice will come from someone who has had their own baby – another mother. She wants advice from personal experience, and preferably recent experience.

Well, I'm happy to stand up and be a face for mental health. Young people who want to die and feel like it is their only option is not okay. I want to help de-stigmatise depression and give hope to those suffering, as well as help the people around them understand what depression feels like.

Almost everyone suffers under the burden of depression at some stage in their lives, either directly or indirectly, but talking about it is taboo. But this isn't some niche illness that we can afford to keep quiet about.

There are celebrities who come out and say they have had mood disorders, such as bipolar or depression. This emphasises that these conditions can and do affect anyone! However, I'm a typical kid, not a superstar or sporting athlete. I haven't won a marathon or set a new world record for anything. I don't have a CD topping the music charts. However, it is an amazing achievement for anyone, regardless of their stature, just to overcome depression. I'm an average kid who went through this and I can still lead a good life. Depression does not define who you are.

When you are in the worst of it, you want to know that you'll come out of it and have relationships; that you will still be able to go out and party. You want to know that you'll be able to continue your studies and hold down a job. As much as everyone wants to be different, they want to be the same. They want to fit in and do all of the stuff that their peers can do.

And I had to tell my story in a book so that others can take it away and read it in private. I had some success talking to parents who were going through it because I'm very candid about my own experience. Not everyone else is. If I go up to a kid and say, 'I understand you are struggling at the moment with depression', there'd be this reaction of, 'Shit, who else knows? What do they think about me? How can this person I barely know have all this information about me?' They'd over-think it.

Outsiders think there must have been a trauma to send me off the edge. But most people I have spoken to who had depression have grown up in happy families with two loving parents. Being in such a fortunate position made me feel more guilty for having these emotions.

Australians are some of the luckiest people on earth. We have clean water; we live in a safe and secure environment; we have plenty to eat. But having these things and the physical comforts most of us enjoy does not mean that you are not allowed to be depressed. You can't compare yourself to others with less material wealth and say, 'I have no right to feel unhappy'. Such emotions can't simply be wished away and suppressing them is not a solution.

People said I just wanted attention, because they couldn't understand it.

There is no scan they can do so society can say, 'Yep, we can see that you've got it'. There is no blood test for it. It's purely symptomatic. So if you are relying on people to tell you that they have depression, you may never find out. How are you going to detect it with no screening process and a general reluctance to talk about it? Even when those affected by depression know there is something wrong, they often don't know where to seek help, let alone how to describe those morbid feelings they don't understand.

Before I started on this book, I took a break overseas. Reliving my story and getting it down on paper was going to be a large undertaking. I wondered to myself, 'Is it even really needed?' After all, everyone in my circle of friends and family already knew what I'd been through. Who else needed to know?

Then two parents came to see me about their son and we sat down to talk for almost two hours. Over the past two years they had travelled a similar road with their son and discovered many of the same things I had, whether it was about not being disheartened when one doctor doesn't click with your child and you need to find one who does, or not sweating over school attendance if your child is safe at home.

mum, i wish i was dead

As we talked, a look came over their faces of relief and hope. They were reasoning that if I could explain in depth what they were going through, and they knew I got through it to the other side, then there is hope for them too. But it is very easy to lose hope.

I'm still young and I remember what it was like in high school. The further you move away from that time, the harder it becomes to recount the experience in a way that is meaningful for those who are there now. Accounts of the traumatic events of adult depression will not have the same relevance to a young person.

Although any episode of depression is traumatic, no matter the age of the person suffering, the challenges are very different for those at varying stages of their life. Adults who have lived longer will have gained a greater perspective.

As an adult, you realise that there is a vast range of future possibilities; teenagers can't imagine life after school. They are so swept up in their closed social world and also feel they have little control over their lives. Teenagers are still developing social skills and establishing support networks. For a teenager coping with depression, it's a whole different obstacle course.

These children are beating themselves up inside. They simply may not know that life can be any different, that these feelings are a part of growing up. Many become so good at putting on a mask that no one has any idea what they are going through. Then you wake up one morning and they aren't there.

I hit rock bottom when I realised I wanted to die. I verbalised it and that's what shocked me. It's very hard to see someone reach that stage.

This isn't a glamorising story. This is just about awareness. It doesn't have all the answers – maybe not even most of the answers, but it was written to give hope.

Even if I could go back and change it all to live a 'normal' life, I wouldn't. I would still choose to live each day and suffer as I did because it has taught me invaluable life lessons and made me the person I am today.

My experiences may have been unique. However, my struggle is all too common …

2

The Happiest Childhood

My version of hurting myself was punching walls. All this physical aggression was held in tight in my upper body. I punched things I could break like the blinds in my room. I broke them many times.

As I got older, when my anger reappeared and I was a lot stronger, I'd punch the wall at home or even at school in sick bay when no one was there to see me. I would breathe out and clench my fists and try to breathe the anger out. Sometimes it was only one punch to a door, or sometimes it was continuous punching as hard as I could into a wall until I literally saw red on the wall. My blood. And even then, it wouldn't stop me.

I didn't feel pain in my hand when I was punching the wall, even though the walls were brick. Afterwards, my hands would be shaking. I'd hit with my hands to the point where I couldn't clench my fists or move my fingers afterwards, that's how much I hurt my hands, because the adrenaline and anger pumping through me blocked all that out. I've still got scars on my knuckles that are only now fading.

Once that short burst of anger was done – and it was extremely short and intense – it was just sadness and tears.

***

'Saba! Saba!' I called as I'd rush excitedly from my mother's car into the assorted jumble of clothes and camping gear of my grandfather's army disposal store. My mother and younger brother, Nathan, followed behind.

The store was in Bondi Junction, the bustling shopping hub of Sydney's eastern suburbs, and my mum would drop us off with my paternal grandfather when she needed some time to go and shop without two little boys underfoot.

We were delighted with the adventure. It was a regular treat that had started when I was young and before Nathan was on the scene. I think we believed that visiting Saba was all about pleasing us, not a convenient break for mum, and Saba always loved having us.

As soon as mum had gone, Saba closed up the store, ignoring his customers, and walked us to the supermarket to buy us some food. We'd stock up on biscuits, cheese and fruit, and take our haul back to his shop. Once there, he would set up a tent right in the middle of his shop for us to eat our supplies in. When we weren't playing in the tent, we would be climbing the ladders around his shop that lead to more merchandise we could play with. It was like being on camp, and no imagination was needed because drinking flasks, cutlery canteens and the whole camping kit surrounded us. It was the perfect stage set for our games.

I don't remember if the 'Closed' sign remained up after our return, but I don't recall ever being interrupted while we set about making camp. It was as if my grandfather's sole purpose in owning the store was to provide a playground for us, and during the hours he spent serving customers, he was only biding his time until his intended patrons, my brother and I, came to visit.

Saba used to come to our house every Tuesday night for dinner, staying on afterwards to babysit while my mum went off to play bridge and dad was at soccer. He also babysat the Saturday nights my parents went out. He would happily eat whatever mum was cooking for us, which was usually pizza or tapas – meals in which she could sneak the vegetables she was keen to feed us. He would also make surprise visits to bring things over for us and he would ring often to see we were okay.

My mother says that family is everything to him and he was just so happy to have, in her words, 'these two gorgeous grandchildren'.

Saba was born in Czechoslovakia and is a Holocaust survivor. He was in a few of the work camps, spent time in Auschwitz and finished the war in Theresienstadt. These were all terrible places, and his experiences here probably explain why he feels that family is so precious. His wife, my grandmother Olga, was born in China to Russian parents. Her family went to Israel and it was there, after the war, that she met him. They had two sons: the elder, Abe, was born in Israel; the younger, Tony (my father), was born once they had immigrated to Australia.

My uncle Abe doesn't have any children so Nathan and I are the only grandchildren on my dad's side. My mother has two brothers but they were late starters in the parenting stakes so my cousins arrived only recently on the scene and are around 20 years younger than me. This made me the first grandchild for both sets of grandparents and meant that I had a huge amount of attention and love lavished on me. There was no competition.

My maternal grandmother, nanna, is like a second mother to me. She is a huge influence in my life. She is only 20 years older than my mum and very youthful. Living close to the water, we would often go to the beach after school and my nanna would join us. She had a huge amount of energy and it was with her that I would go exploring the rock pools, looking at all the crabs, and then head off on rock-climbing expeditions. She'd be the one digging tunnels in the sand and jumping in the waves with us. My mum says that she was like a child herself when she was with us and she related to us really well. I loved the beach. It's a place where I always felt relaxed and free. The beach was a major part of my life growing up.

Whenever we wanted to stay over with nanna and poppa, we did. Nathan and I would sleep next to their bed on the floor. Mum would say: 'You're going on holidays to nanna and poppa's', and we'd both get really excited. It was only years later that I discovered that she sold it to us as a holiday, but it was actually that she and dad were going away for the weekend. Not that we would have felt abandoned because it really was a holiday to be over at their place.

I spent a lot of time with nanna when I was young, almost every moment I could. When we were at her place, she'd let us get away with everything. Nathan and I would ask if we could build a cubby house and she'd agree, as long as we used only one mattress. Of course, we completely disregarded that instruction and used every single pillow in the house, including all those on the beds and the lounges. The whole house would be turned upside down as we'd build our fortress. We used absolutely everything and nanna never got angry. I used to think that I had cleverly convinced my nanna to allow me to do what I wanted – that I was a skilled negotiator who had concealed the true extent of my intentions. Looking back on it, she must have known what we were up to. She just enjoyed seeing us happy. Every memory I have of her is a good one.

Saying 'memory' makes it sound as if my nanna was only part of that idyllic childhood. Actually, she's been around for me until this day and I still see her each week. Every time I have needed someone, she has always been there. I will ring her and say, 'Let's go out for lunch or a coffee'. When something is troubling me, I will seek her counsel.

My nanna is possibly the most empathetic and selfless person I have known. She will always put others before herself and drop everything to do things for other people. Both her parents died when she was quite young, as did her brother. She was orphaned at 17, before she married. Her sister, the last remaining immediate family member, died from lung cancer when I was 11. Unfortunately, nanna has suffered from the same affliction and after two bouts of lung cancer herself, she has been left with only one lung. For someone used to doing so much, her physical ill health has really reduced what she is capable of. The woman who always asked: 'If you need anything, just let me know?', still makes the same offer. Only now we know it means that if you tell her what you need, she'll organise my poppa to do it!

When things started going wrong for me, my nanna played a big part in keeping me safe and helping me on the road to recovery, but that comes later …

My poppa's parents were still alive when I was young, so I was lucky enough to have great-grand parents and they lived close to us too. My great-grandfather was a terrific storyteller, so visits to his house were enchanting. He was Scottish and his stories were no doubt enhanced by his wonderfully thick and exotic accent. We would have a regular routine where, as soon as we arrived at their house, Nathan and I would be officially measured and our growing heights recorded, we'd feed the birds, and then we'd be rewarded with chocolate.

With so much love and attention from my grandparents, you'd almost think that they were making up for absent parents – but that wasn't the case. As far as my parents were concerned, I had much more than many children can hope for. My mother was completely devoted to her children and enjoyed our company. She would, however, have been grateful for the additional support she received from our grandparents because, for much of the time my father was at work. That's not to say my father wasn't devoted to us too. It's just that it was important to him to provide for all our financial needs and that meant working six days a week and long hours into the night, which kept him away until after we'd had dinner and often already gone to bed. With hindsight, I realise he was busy starting his new law firm; however, as a young kid I didn't understand why he had to be absent.

Lucky for her I was an easy baby and a fairly easy child. She speaks glowingly about my textbook behaviour. 'Adam dropped his first feed of the morning by six weeks and was sleeping through the night by eight weeks'. Apparently, that's a big deal because, as any harried young parents will tell you, a night of uninterrupted sleep where they don't have to get up to a crying baby is the holy grail of early parenthood.

My mum also says that I was mindful of not imposing myself on my parents, so for example when I woke in the morning I wouldn't call out for them or scream. They would come to my bedroom to find me playing with my mobile – not a phone but the toys that dangle above a baby's cot – or just sitting up in bed and amusing myself. She says she could go and take a shower, sit me down in front of a mirror, and I would quietly bide my time. I think I was a pretty contented child.

Also forming the network of support was what I like to think of as our 'extended family', a group of family friends with whom we are still close today. They were really my parents' friends, but they all had children around our age and because we socialised together the kids all became friends. There are probably about seven families all up, and today the children range in age from about 16 to 28. We often went on holidays together, so any vacation could include four or five families with more than a dozen children in tow. There was always someone around your age or who shared your interest and was happy to play with you. We now know each other very well and will always be a part of each other's lives in one way or another. They are more like cousins, and we still get together as families for the occasional dinner and special events.

With all this love and me being the perfect child, how could anything go wrong? Well, maybe I wasn't so perfect.

Apparently, I was not so good at sharing my toys. Is any kid? At day care, I used to love playing with the toy animals. I remember walking in one day and one of the other children ran up to me and said: 'Adam, Adam, I've been looking after your animals for you and I haven't let anyone touch them'. So even then, the other kids knew that I thought of these as mine, and a no-go area for anyone else.

If I could feel that proprietorial about the kindy toys, you can bet I was even more determined about keeping my own things for myself, and prize among my possessions was my Lego. I could spend hours with those blocks and everyone knew that the perfect present for me for any occasion was something to add to my ever-growing collection. If I was sent to my room for any transgression, I went quietly, happy to be alone and constructing. It was hardly a punishment to me and my parents would have to come and get me out before I would ask to be released.

Like a lot of kids, I also felt most comfortable with routine and didn't like any last-minute changes to the planned events of the day. As she dropped me off at kindy, my mum could tell me that, come the afternoon, we'd be going to the hairdressers or some other appointment, and I'd be cool with that when she arrived to pick me up at the end of the day. But should she not mention the appointment until I was in the car, expecting to go home, I would lose it. I didn't like having anything sprung on me.

Perhaps I was a little more rigid than most about that. When I knew what was happening in advance, even if it hadn't been my choice, I had no problem with falling into line and being compliant. I just needed to know the rules or the structure and not have that change on me without notice. My mum learned that if she kept me advised and didn't reorganise things at the last moment, I was much easier to deal with.

Once, at a friend's house, when I was about four years old, we were talking about sleepovers, and I must have asked the question, 'Can I sleep over here tonight?' 'Yes, yes,' my mother said, probably trying to brush me off and with little real intention that she would be leaving me behind that night, guessing I would have forgotten in the hours before we departed. However, when my mum went to go, I had a tantrum because she had promised I could sleep there. In the end, she relented because she realised that she had made a commitment.

Parents often say things they don't mean for the sake of keeping the peace and their children happy. I believe in sticking by your word, and that has been something important in our family. Better the truth at the start and then you can reconcile yourself to it, than to create false expectations, dash people's hopes, and ultimately undermine their trust. Children may look like they are buzzing around with thoughts flitting in and out of their minds, but they remember what they're told and the promises made to them.

My need for organisation and being in control of my timetable played out when I got to primary school. As soon as I was given any work to do, I had to do it straightaway. If it came to recess or lunchtime and I hadn't completed the tasks we'd been assigned, I'd stay in the classroom until it was finished. We were generally given our homework for the week on Mondays, and as soon as I'd get home on Monday afternoon, I had to get it all over and done with. I wanted to have mum by my side so that if I had to write anything, she could check that my spelling and sentence structure was okay. It was not just important to finish the work, it had to be done as well as I could do it.

Maybe the additional motivation for all this was that I liked to please, whether it was my parents, my friends or my teachers. I had a sense of myself as a 'good boy' and I was always treated as such, so I didn't want to disappoint. That attitude carried on almost until the end of primary school.

I did really well at school and enjoyed getting good results in my exams. Not that I studied because I didn't know how to do that. I didn't have any sporting ability but my natural ability was in the academic side of my life. That's where I received acknowledgement for doing well in my exams. No one pushed me to do well. It was an internal pressure I placed on myself.

Although I was academic, I still knew how to have fun. Come time for recess and lunch, or even after school care, that was my chance to be with my friends and muck around. I probably had more friendships with girls than with the other boys, and have always been drawn to females from a young age. Whether that's the result of the close relationships I have with my mother and grandmother, I'm not sure, but girls are more empathetic, nurturing and kind. I wasn't consciously aware of it at the time, but I did have more female friends. However, there has always been a couple of very close best male friends, the kind whom I could build Lego, play video games and have sleepovers with.

All told, I was a happy kid who enjoyed and excelled at school. So what was the downside, because there always has to be one? It wasn't the classroom, where I had friends and was liked by teachers. It was on the sports field.

3

Boy Stuff, Ball Games and Bullying

This is why I hate Sunday morning. It should be fun, since it's the weekend and the one day of the week when my dad is around. Like most of the dads in our circle of friends, he loves to play and watch soccer. He would make the time to go and see my brother play and I joined a local team so that I could spend more time with him too.

I know dad made as much time as possible for us. He did his best to balance up his work commitments and his family time. Dad came to every single one of my school camps and was always at the major events – every sports carnival, every award night and all the parent-teacher interviews. As a kid I didn't see those events as important, possibly due to my attention being focused on my friends rather than the surrounding adults. Nonetheless, I wanted a reason for us to be together on a regular basis and to have something we could bond over like I saw him and Nathan having.

Here I was in the under 10Cs, which gives you a sense that we weren't really a group of top-notch players. Even then, I felt like I was definitely the weak link, letting the side down at every game. I just wasn't very good at any kind of sport, and team sports were the worst because, on top of personal failure was the added pressure of not disappointing the other members of the team. Because soccer was that meeting point for building a rapport with my father, that made my poor performance at the game a triple insult.

Now my dad never made me feel bad about how I played, but I knew it was a big deal for him. I could see how much pleasure it gave him to be at Nathan's games and see his younger son be covered in glory. In fact, my dad was quite good on the sidelines, which is more than I can say about the other parents who were so competitive that they were not above yelling abuse at the kids on the field. It really turned me off team sport and I very quickly came to despise soccer.

Somehow playing sport at school wasn't quite as bad and I fared much better, often being the first to be picked for a side or captaining the team. It was still competitive, but in a much more friendly way. I wasn't being judged or ridiculed by the parents and the whole spirit was much less serious. There were also the games we would play at lunchtime, which were about having fun more than anything else.

The weekend games of soccer in winter and cricket in summer were part of the ritual among our family friends. There was an expectation that I would be involved because all the kids did it, and especially because I was the oldest child. The first-borns in the group played and excelled at sport. Even conversation among the guys revolved around playing or watching sport, and I felt embarrassed to contribute to the discussions.

Unlike me, Nathan was always very sporty and sporting victory came easily to him. I definitely resented that. Here I was, the older brother, and my younger sibling was excelling at something that I found difficult. It wasn't just in sport that this difference emerged. We are like chalk and cheese. He was very slim and could eat anything he wanted without care, and I was becoming chubby – not the ideal physique for sporting prowess. I had to watch everything I ate and it didn't feel fair.

Whatever I chose to eat, my dad would have a go at me. In retrospect, I think this was because my dad had always struggled with his weight and didn't want me to suffer as he did. We would often clash over food. Not that our diet at home was unhealthy. Mum always made sure that afternoon snacks were raw vegetables or fruit. It's not like I was always eating cake and chocolates. But it was obvious that whatever I was consuming was turning to fat on me and was simply sliding off my brother. He was skinny; I was fat.

While weekend sport had turned into a nightmare, Saturday swimming was still a joy. For a start, this wasn't a team sport so I was only ever competing with myself to get better. I preferred the solo sports because I wasn't the one letting the team down and I didn't need to rely on other people to succeed. I loved swimming and I was very good at it.

All the family friends would get together for swimming lessons but my father was usually not there. He would turn up at the end of the day, but that wasn't the same as having him there, watching me at the one sport in which I excelled. I really did miss having him around. If he hadn't been working and was down at the pool or the beach with us, I think that we could have enjoyed each other's company. But as Sunday was his only free day, it made our interactions over the dreaded soccer field more intense and fraught. This was our only opportunity during the week to hang out with each other and it wasn't an activity in which we shared an interest. However, I was still at that stage when I wanted desperately to please so I didn't see a way around it. I wasn't capable of saying that I wanted to spend time with him but I wanted to do something else. After all, I was only 10. Maybe there was also an element of, 'this is your special thing with Nathan. I want to have a special, but different, connection with you too', especially because his time was so precious.

During our childhood, I craved my father's attention. It wasn't only Saturday swimming lessons where I felt his absence. School holidays would start with the three of us heading off and dad joining us some time later or maybe catching up on the weekend and then heading back to the office on the Monday. He took his role as breadwinner for the family very seriously. He felt my mum was very capable and competent, and that he wasn't missed. This couldn't have been further from the truth. He was showing us his love by giving us everything but his time. Only now can I appreciate and actually understand how much he did for us.

As a child, all I could tell was that I was missing out on something I wanted. My dad missed out as well, because he didn't realise that we wanted him for more than his pay cheque. He could have been having fun with us instead of slaving away in the office. We wanted him with us more than we could say.

mum, i wish i was dead

Towards the end of Year 4 in primary school, I did start to feel conscious about the way I looked. Before then I was completely indifferent to it. I stopped feeling comfortable even going to the beach or swimming and when I did go, I'd resort to wearing a rash vest to cover up as much as I could.

Always a 'solid' child, I had become quite chubby. There was some bullying about my appearance, and in particular when I started wearing glasses. I was teased about being fat and also for getting on well with girls. There were days when I came home upset about being the butt of these unkind comments, although at the time I believed I was shrugging them off and that the bullying was having no lasting effect on me.

The weight I was piling on was another point of conflict for me with my brother Nathan. He didn't do anything wrong, but I was jealous of his natural abilities at sport for which he was always praised, and the fact that he could eat whatever he wanted and remain slim. It wasn't his fault, but I could see it every day at the dinner table; I would eat the same meal as him and put on weight whereas he wouldn't. Because my weight was becoming a real issue, that really grated on me. It was in my face.

I should say that Nathan never gave me a hard time about my weight. He was never rude to me. Of course we did fight over things, but it was the usual stupid stuff that brothers do. It was very funny because I was big and strong, and he was always the little one, so my parents presumed that I was giving Nathan grief.

We used to watch the wrestling together on TV and we'd pretend to wrestle. No one got hurt, but Nathan would 'put it on', pretending that I had done him an injury. Even when we were just watching the screen, Nathan would start screaming out of the blue and crying, so that my parents would come running to his assistance. Even though I knew that he was faking it, I would get into trouble.

One day, when I was about 12, we were watching TV and the same routine started up with Nathan screaming blue murder. Both parents came running to the room, demanding to know what I had done to him and telling me that Nathan was so much smaller than me and I had to be careful with him.

All the while, Nathan was hiding under a blanket with his face covered, sobbing. I had to defend myself so I said, 'he's not upset, look', and I whipped the blanket off him. He had the biggest smile on his face. Ever since then they weren't as quick to believe him.

So I think we had a very typical sibling rivalry. I knew I could never even compete when it came to basketball and soccer, but with all the family friends, I never tried to fit in that way. I left that to Nathan. I always got on better with the girls because they didn't want to talk about sport all the time. I found them much more interesting.

I loved watching the wrestling on TV, even though I knew it was faked – just like Nathan's performances. I definitely grew up watching a lot of wrestling! Even though we had TV and we had Game Boys and Nintendo 64s, we didn't have the Internet. It wasn't really around, so afternoons after school were much more social. We would have afternoon tea with mum or at my grandmother's place, and we'd talk about the day.

While I don't recall being teased each day at school, one child in particular did bully me. Ironically, this was a kid who I thought would have my back and always look out for me. He never said anything to my face or put me down publicly, but he did exclude me from activities in the playground. He changed school eventually so that nasty experience came to an end. However, I never liked bullies and would intervene if I saw them being cruel to anyone else. I have a strong sense about what is just and am troubled when people are unfairly treated.

There was another kid who was a bully in general but not to me in particular. We always used to play handball at school and, one day, a kid in the year above us asked to join our game. Whoever owned the tennis ball we were using was the controller of the game and made the rules. This day, it was the bully's ball and he said 'no' to the kid.

'Well, that's fine,' I said, and I took my tennis ball and went off with the kid, just the two of us, and we played together. He was so appreciative that he told his parents and they told my parents. When my parents asked me about the incident, I had completely forgotten it had happened. But they were happy to have been complimented on their son's behaviour.

From a young age, I've always been anti-bullying. I don't like excluding people. Whenever bullying occurred, I was never confrontational; instead I would simply remove myself from the situation.

Perhaps I was good with kids socially because I was usually in a composite class at school, so I had to deal with children of different ages and abilities. There could be up to three Year groups combined, and I might be one of only six kids in my age group. We were generally the ones doing well academically, and there were mainly girls in that group. Sometimes I was the only boy from my Year in the classroom. I seemed never to be in a class of just my Year.

I always had friends and my marks were good. My parents will say I was a happy child, and gave them very little cause for concern. But about Year 5, things started to change.

Looking back, it's hard to know what the first signs were. I was certainly right in the middle of it, and even I had no idea what was happening to me. Yes, it was around the time that I was becoming aware and insecure about my physical appearance. Was it just the start of adolescence and the beginning of hormonal changes?

If my mum is asked to pinpoint it, she'll say that one of the big red warning flags came the day when I refused to go to school.

4

'My Heart is Black, My Body is Full of Anger'

My mother started to get the feeling that things weren't so good for me at school. She says that she felt I was on my own and not playing with anyone. Unbeknown to me, she went to speak to the teachers and they reassured her that I had lots of friends and that everyone liked me.

'Even if he is sitting on his own, everyone who walks past him would have a chat or say hello', they told her. 'Even when he goes to the library, it's his choice to be away from his friends, not because people aren't including him.'

However, the teacher I had had for a couple of years in a row took my mother aside and confided in her. 'I shouldn't be showing you this yet', she said, handing my mum one of my latest maths tests. 'Usually Adam gets over 90. On this test he got just 60. I have to ask you, is something upsetting Adam? Is something wrong?'

From a star performer, I'd plummeted to someone who was barely scraping a pass. My mum knew that it wasn't because I wasn't capable, and the mark would have been further evidence that the child who had caused her no concern to date was taking a turn for the worse.

At this time, I started to refuse to go to school. In the beginning, it was on Mondays that I chose not to attend. I couldn't face the return to school after the break of the weekend. At home, my family would say that I had

'Monday-itis'. It wasn't every Monday I didn't go to school, but near enough to every one. And then my phobia of school progressed so that I wouldn't go on other days of the week as well.

My mother recalls one day I came home and complained about being teased and demanded not to be taken to school again. Things must have been coming to a head before this, because I was coming home in the afternoons and going straight to bed, sometimes sleeping for four hours. My usual morning routine was also being abandoned as I refused to get dressed when I'd wake up.

I never gave a reason for not wanting to go to school and I don't remember being asked. In truth, I don't believe I knew what the reason was. A psychologist I was taken to see because of my refusal to attend school asked me, 'if you had three wishes, what would they be?' My response was, 'Not to have to go to school, to be thinner, and to have less rules at home'. I was about 10 or 11 at the time.

Rather than try to discover why I had developed a reluctance to attend classes, my mother was being advised just to get me straight back to school, at all costs. But she simply couldn't. I was a big boy. How could she drag me against my will, kicking and screaming from the house, into a car, and then out of it at the other end? Much less, how could she even get me into my uniform? She was told, 'Take him to school in his pyjamas if he won't dress for school'. She never even tried because she knew it wasn't going to happen. The psychologist I went to focused on getting me to school.

Luckily, my mum started to see a psychologist, someone to help her personally with this developing dilemma. She'd actually been 'shopping around' for a psychologist for me, but this woman said she didn't see young people in her practice. Instead, why doesn't mum come around and make an appointment for herself? Luckily she did. The psychologist actually taught my mum a lot of tools she could use in dealing with me and challenged her thinking. It has turned out to be a valuable relationship and, to this day, my mum still visits this woman when she has any concerns.

Mum also started to trust her own gut feeling that was telling her to back off and stop putting pressure on me. When she did that, things began easing up. She realised that it didn't really make a difference to anybody whether I was home. She did feel, however, that I probably needed to get out of the house, so she'd try and find diversions and excuses to drag me out the front door. If Nathan was playing basketball, she'd say let's go and watch. Sometimes I'd join her; other times I'd ask to be left alone. She wouldn't fight my decision. As she says now, you have to pick your battles and I was safe at home.

Ultimately, she knew I'd make the right decision, whether it was going to a family function or turning up to school when I was ready. Some mornings she would come into my room and say, 'Adam, school?'

'No, I don't feel like going today.'

'Okay,' she'd respond, and turn around and walk out. Next thing she'd know, I'd be dressed and downstairs, ready to go off to school.

Mum says, 'I was told someone like Adam knows right from wrong, and the more you tell him, it's just bombarding him and going around in his head.' She learned to trust my judgement, and it was a tactic that worked.

Big picture-wise, I knew I was meant to be at school. When I stopped being told that I had to go, I slowly started to come around a bit. At first, my mum would say, 'If you can go to school for an hour in the morning, that would be great.' So I did. That would build up to staying until lunchtime, and then I would go for full days.

By the end of Year 5, the school refusal was sorted, and things finished on a high note for me. I was voted in as a leader for the approaching final year of primary school. To outsiders, it could have looked as if everything was back on track. Even the psychologist I was seeing told my mother that it may have been a one-off incident, and my mum certainly hoped that was the case. In the back of her mind, though, she thought there was something else wrong, but she didn't know what it was. 'We've got him back to school, but what caused the refusal in the first place?' she wondered.

My mother blames herself for not being a good listener and for glossing over any of my complaints. She'll tell you that she is the kind of person who just gets on with things; if something happens that you don't like, you put it behind you and move on.

In contrast, I would blow everything out of proportion. I could come home from school and say things like, 'A teacher did this to me today or something happened with a friend of mine that really upset me'.

Her response would be, 'Tomorrow is another day. Everyone will have forgotten about it by then'.

mum, i wish i was dead

When we discuss it now, she says that I probably needed to talk about it more and she was too dismissive. She believed that there was a lot I wanted to tell her but she wasn't open to hearing it because we deal with problems differently. But I honestly don't think I knew what was happening to me. I simply didn't have the words to describe my problems to anyone and I didn't even understand what was going on myself.

That led to a huge frustration for me. I was like a volcano, ready to erupt. It just kept building … building … building, and then suddenly it had to come out. So during my primary school years from around the age of nine, even before my refusal to attend school, and into high school, there would be periods of rage. They were probably dismissed as tantrums when I was younger, and my parents may have consoled themselves that I would grow out of them at some stage. However, as I grew older and stronger, the outbursts became more violent.

When the psychologist I saw asked me to tell her what negatives there were about me, the one thing I told her was, 'I have a really bad temper that I bottle up. When it comes out, it becomes ranting and raving.' When asked about my positive traits, I was not so quick to answer, having to think for a while of any. And then it was, 'I'm kind, good at building Lego and good at listening'.

With the anger, I was trying to suppress whatever feelings I had and keep functioning, and then I would just explode. It cost me a huge amount of energy to face the world as if nothing was wrong. I managed to keep it together when I was at school, but as soon as I got home, I would barricade myself in my bedroom and start throwing things around the room.

The tension would build up to the point where I was always moody and snappy, but never with my friends, only at home. I was leading this double life. Whenever my parents had any interaction with my school, they'd be told how wonderful I was and what a delight to teach. My parents joked that they should have built our house in the school grounds so that I exhibited that behaviour at home.

My mum knew that I wasn't being naughty, but she was frightened about the anger I was expressing and the fact that I might cause myself harm. She could live with the broken cupboard doors and the torn blinds. The furniture was the least of her worries. There was no lock on my door, but I would manage to jam it closed so no one could get inside. I did this as much to be alone, as to spare the rest of the family my outbursts. It wasn't a show for them, and I desperately didn't want to hurt or upset them. I think I've spent my whole life trying to please and be good, and I could never physically hurt anyone. I could, however, see that I was causing them serious worry, and that didn't please me, but I was powerless to do anything about it.

From the other side of the door, my mum says that it sounded crazy inside my bedroom. She'd beg me to let her in. 'No, no, go away,' I'd demand. She learned over time that if I was very bad, it was better for her to leave me alone and things would settle down much more quickly.

As soon as my rage was spent, I'd burst into tears and begin sobbing. Things would eventually calm down after I had cried out all my frustration and it had poured out of me. I'd 'unlock' my door, and my mum knew that things were alright again. After one episode, when I was 10, mum came into my room to ask what was wrong. This is what I said: 'My heart is black. My body is full of anger. And I wish I was dead.' This was years before I had heard of or understood the words 'depression' and 'suicide'. It was the only way I knew how to verbally describe the intense, unknown feelings I had.

When my mother had sought out professional advice about me, people had offered her band-aid solutions, implying that my issues could be easily resolved. Many people said that I was just after attention. I think she realised at this point that there was a deeper, underlying problem.

My darkest moments were usually at night before I fell asleep. During the day, I could distract myself by watching TV or playing. I could stop myself from thinking. As soon as there was silence and quiet, that's when all the thoughts would come tumbling in.

It was not one or two thoughts, but hundreds, if not thousands – all at the same time and all negative. It was unimaginably hard to deal with and it happened every day, relentlessly. I was over-thinking and re-thinking events that had happened, thinking about future possibilities and catastrophising everything. I had no control over my thoughts.

In those moments, I remember imagining something horrific happening to me: a plane crash or the death of someone close to me. I toyed with these ideas, not because I feared the worst, but because such a scenario would give justification to why I felt so bad. I thought that if something terrible happened to me, people would start believing me when I said I was unhappy and understand my pain.

I thought that a personal tragedy would explain my condition. I wanted other people to 'get' why I felt that way. Adults couldn't understand my pain, let alone people my own age. I don't think even my family, who supported me, really understood. How could they? I couldn't explain it to myself. All I knew was how bad I felt and how desperate I was for it to stop.

The frustration of not being able to make the pain go away made me very angry. I would become verbally abusive and violent with all this physical anger that would just build up. But I only expressed the violence against inanimate objects and myself. I never wanted to hurt anyone, ever.

I would destroy my room, rip the door off its hinges and flip my bed upside down. I would punch holes in doors and I would punch the wall until it turned red with my blood. I would bang my head against the wall because I wanted to try and silence the black thoughts.

Just as I would never lash out and hit anyone, I could never intentionally cause emotional hurt to others. I'm sure they were anxious enough about my wellbeing, but I wouldn't bring them any further suffering. I think that's the reason I didn't kill myself. I knew what my death would do to my family, especially my mother and my nanna. I knew that they loved me and were fighting for me to get better.

Strangely, I did feel that I was their biggest burden and I thought their lives would be easier without me, but they constantly told me how much they loved me. The thought of how much my death would hurt them was the *only* thing that kept me alive.

I did, however, imagine my death. I used to sit there and wonder if anyone outside my family would even bother to turn up for the funeral. Would any of my friends be there? I felt so empty that I believed no one would even notice that I was gone.

I was feeling sad and angry, and felt that no one understood me. Even I didn't understand me. I found myself confiding in one of my closest friends – my grandparent's dog Windsor. Windsor had been around since I was born, so we had grown up together. He had been a fixture my entire life.

One of my greatest consolations as a child had been animals. I love animals and always feel comfortable around them. We were Zoo Friends at

Taronga Park Zoo. This meant that we visited almost every month. It was a great trek out there and a full, big day. I'm always calm around animals, whether they are large animals such as horses, or small like snakes. Animals were a big part of my life.

Windsor was a little fox terrier. We said that he had nine lives because he fell down the stairs twice, and had been hit by a car twice and lost one of his legs. He'd been mauled by a dog four times his size, but he kept surviving these disasters. I spent so much time at my grandparents' house and Windsor was always there. As I grew older, when I slept over at my grandparents I was given my own bedroom, and Windsor would sleep at the end of my bed. When my grandparents came in, he'd growl at them, or anyone coming near me. He protected me. He never harmed me in any way.

One afternoon, I caught the bus to my grandparents' place and Windsor wasn't at the door to jump up and greet me. My nanna had one of her friends over, so I retreated to another room and began to play with my Lego. I heard snippets of their conversation, including the words, 'What are we going to tell Adam?' After the friend departed, I started to question where Windsor was and became more frantic and upset. 'Where's Windsor? Where's Windsor?'

Nanna sat me down and said that they had to send him away to a farm because he was very sick, but in the country he would be very well looked after and safe. He'd be able to run around with his friends. I was distressed that I hadn't been able to say goodbye, and I sobbed for hours. It is the first really upsetting experience that I can recall from my childhood.

I believed nanna at the time, and it wasn't until much later – an embarrassingly long time later – that I realised Windsor had actually died then. He had been very sick, suffering a lot of pain, and he was starting to nip at people. My grandparents had to put him down. At the time, as a 10-year-old, all I knew was that he was gone. My best friend was gone like that, without any explanation, without a goodbye.

***

My grandparents were not the only family members who provided emotional support to me as a young boy. At times when I was quite bad, either refusing to go to school or having bouts of sadness, my mother would enlist the help of others.

mum, i wish i was dead

At the time, I was unaware of her role in arranging the 'handrails' to help me on my path. It was her invisible hand that tried to guide me away from the depths of despair. Just as well that I was ignorant of her involvement because I'm sure I would have resented it and rebelled against it.

One person conscripted by my mum was her brother David. She would phone him when I was bad and needed someone to get me out of the house. He would then call me and ask me to hang out with him.

My Uncle David was into aquatic life, whether that was in the fresh air and by the seaside, or neatly housed in an aquarium. One of our projects was installing a fish tank at home, and we would make regular excursions to the fish shop to stock the tank. Another favourite activity was to go down to the harbour and hire a sailing boat or a kayak, get some food, and sail or row to one of the beaches where we could have our lunch. We'd just spend the day together having a boys' own adventure.

It got me into the fresh air, down to the water, and I was exercising without even realising it. These outings were always fun and there was no pressure or any emotional discussion. We were very matter-of-fact, just dealing with the task at hand. David and I got on very well and I always looked forward to being with him.

It was always David who called me. Mum could never have convinced me to ring him. Anything she suggested I do when I was in a gloomy mood would be refused. For a start, I didn't have the energy to do anything myself. The other reason was that I needed to hear from other people that they wanted to be with me. I didn't want anyone to agree to spend time with me because I had asked them.

When I was down in the dumps, I felt like I was a burden. My perception was that others didn't want to be around me. And I also didn't want to inconvenience anyone by calling them up and asking them to keep me company. Surely they would only say 'yes' out of a sense of pity or guilt, whereas if they made contact with me first, it must mean they actually were keen to see me.

***

Even though I had many sad and painful times in those early years, it may sound strange but my memories of primary school are mostly good ones.

It's fair to say that I loved primary school, in spite of the school refusal. Primary school is easy. There's not a lot of pressure or dire consequences for not doing things.

Towards the end of primary school, girls and boys were starting to show their interest in each other. I was putting on weight and didn't feel included in all that. That's the time I became concerned about my body and didn't know what to do about it. Conversations around who liked whom left me feeling excluded. For all this, it was a very sad day when primary school ended. I wasn't looking forward to high school.

It sort of hits you that you've spent years with these kids, and when you are young having been at school from the ages of 6 to 12, that's half your life that you've known them all. You've seen them every day and all day. And even when you'd get home, you'd sit down and call them on the landline – we didn't have mobile phones in those days – or your parents would be driving you out to meet them. The friendships I'd developed made it hard to say goodbye to that.

We were all going to different high schools. A lot of the kids were going to schools where they already knew people. I'd already lost quite a few good friends in Year 4 when they had moved to new schools and I had been left to forge new and stronger friendships.

I was going to a high school where I would know no one. What was worse, having been a child who always sought out the company of girls, my destination was a private school that was only for boys.

I don't remember ever having a good day there.

5

Art Therapy

One of the advantages of refusing to go to school was that I got to meet some interesting people who visited the house during the day. One of these was to have a lasting impact on my life.

My mum was involved in the school P&C and was organising a fundraising trivia night. Another parent at the school, also on the organising committee, came over to our place to work on the event. Newly arrived from South Africa, Michelle was keen to get involved in the local community and this was probably one of the ways she thought she might do that.

Like any curious 10-year-old, I wanted to get in on the action, and offered to help the group. Michelle would certainly have been aware that I was having problems because I wasn't at school when I should have been, and I think my mum may have let her know that things were not so good for me.

An artist herself, Michelle also taught art, and I'm not sure if it was her suggestion or my mum's that I go to her for classes, one-on-one. When my mum mentioned the idea to me, I was very happy to go. It turns out that I was her first student in Australia.

Michelle is an incredibly empathetic woman and we clicked straightaway. She just 'gets' kids, and talking with her was wonderful.

Once a week – during the day if I wasn't going to school or afternoons if I was – my mum would drop me off at Michelle's home. We'd walk up her driveway and there she'd be sitting in her garage turned studio, and she'd walk out to greet us. The garage door would be open to the sunshine and had a view to the ocean.

Mum would leave me with Michelle and together we'd go up to her house and have afternoon tea and biscuits. Unlike my modern home, Michelle's place was a curiosity, small and full of fascinating stuff. There were artworks on every wall, books spilling from shelves, and we'd have our tea from mismatched china in the dining area off her tiny kitchen. Michelle's home was a wonderful Bohemian jumble. It was very exotic for me.

Over time I became more familiar with the place and I'd go up to the kitchen and head straight for the pantry where I could help myself to whatever I wanted to eat. Or, if I felt like a hot chocolate, Michelle and I would make it together. Our little shared meal finished, we would head back to the studio for the class. It was a very comforting ritual.

The studio was organised chaos. It was crammed with the most extraordinary assortment of art materials, reference books, and strange and inexplicable objects that might prove to be inspiration for works or implements for applying paint. Every surface was covered, and pictures were affixed to the rare patches of exposed wall. Magazines were piled high; there were cups full of pencils, crayons and felt-tipped pens; and a rusty, teddy-bear cake tin. Wherever you looked there was an abundance of objects.

It was a tiny space and not much more than six feet high. You could barely stand up and clear the ceiling. Because of this, Michelle joked that: 'When you reach a certain height, you've learned all that I can teach you.' Michelle still refers to it as her cave, and were it not for the expansive view of open sky when the door is up, it would definitely feel subterranean.

Michelle would lay the studio table as if it were for a meal instead of an art class. She'd put a lot of material out so I could make my own choice about what I wanted to use, and I never knew from week to week what I'd be doing. For her it was not so much about the finished artwork I would make, but the process I chose to get there.

At the start, I would only draw with lead pencil, refusing to use any colour or paint. I felt there wasn't any colour I could use because I wasn't joyful. The images I drew were from my imagination of robots, monsters, action figures and guns. I was very stuck in my ways, doing only what I wanted to do and nothing else.

Michelle tried gently to encourage me to move on from my pencil drawings, but I would keep saying, 'What can I paint? What can I represent?' I put up a lot of resistance to trying new things and I didn't want to draw from life because that's what photos are for. Realising that I found it difficult to create images, Michelle decided to focus on a technical exercise. 'Let's make our own colours,' she would say. That was my big transition from monochrome grey to colour.

She had a lot of pigments from the earth and flowers, which we mixed together. We'd take a pigment from a bit of rock, grind that up and add water. It was quite physical. We experimented by adding oil and egg to bind the pigment together.

Through the process of experimenting with our own colours, textures, patterns and brush strokes in my artworks, I started to become more adventurous.

The first painting I made with our newly created colours was a self-portrait. I had to take a small mirror and look at sections of my face and then translate it to paper, piece by piece. There was a message in the way I was instructed to do this. I think Michelle was trying to teach me that people are made up of all these different parts. She liked to have a message in her lessons.

We spent a long, long time on that portrait and it was very slow work. I didn't enjoy that at all. Michelle had to metaphorically hold my hand through the whole process. It was so difficult because I didn't like to reflect on myself. I'm sure Michelle was trying to get me to be more accepting of who I was.

The self-portrait was the first to go home as a gift for my mother. From then on there was an avalanche of paintings that came home, which were then displayed around the house. I was very proud of my efforts and visitors always said nice things about them. It gave me another area in which to do well. One of my teachers who saw these artworks even commissioned me to do a piece for her. My mother grumbled that it was a better version than the one we had at home and she was envious!

My mum says now that she knew what kind of emotional state I was in by the works I brought home. When I was well, my artwork was full of colour. Then suddenly artwork was coming home that was black, white and red. These were the colours when I was slipping. Both my mum and Michelle commented on it. It was interesting how the colours would change. When I'm good, there's a lot of blue.

Once we'd had the colour breakthrough, it went on from there. Michelle would always push very gently without me needing to say 'no'. She was very good at reading me and knowing when to introduce new techniques without applying any pressure. We'd talk while we'd paint alongside each other, each involved in our own pursuit. If I were drawing in pencil she'd be drawing in colour to show how it could be used.

It was quite funny because over the years she wanted me to get that education in art: read art books or go to a gallery. I never wanted to do any of that, only because I enjoyed what I was doing and the history didn't matter. I was never interested in going to any other art teacher or even in studying art at school. I see art as an interactive thing with someone I care about.

It's never been a desire for me to see art. I'd rather be doing it. I'm sure Michelle taught me something by showing me examples of other styles. She took me through every possible form of art: pencil drawing, flower pressing, bleach on black paper, water colours, clay sculpting, different tools, abstract, realist, and using your hands and not just brushes. It reached a point that I would spill coffee on an artwork and incorporate that into the picture. It allowed me to not be the perfectionist I was and I could let go. You can use anything and I very rarely used a paintbrush to paint.

From being very cautious and rigid at the beginning, I'd become a risk-taker with my art.

I always felt comfortable at Michelle's and was excited to go. I never said 'no' to art class and there were times when I'd say 'no' to almost everything else; times when I didn't want to see people, I didn't want to go to the shops, I didn't want to do anything.

I didn't have any interest in art before going to see Michelle and my mother had encouraged me to go purely for therapy, although she would never have said that to me. And it was great therapy, though Michelle would be the first to tell you that she isn't an art therapist. She's an artist, an historian and an educator.

We spoke a lot during the lesson, and the art was somehow incidental. It was almost like something we were doing with our hands while we were really having a conversation.

We had a very special relationship. Michelle made a contract with me that she wouldn't report anything I said in class back to my mum unless there was something that caused her alarm. There was a sense of confidentiality and trust. I'd talk about my family and the struggles at home and at school. My mum would have known that I was speaking openly with Michelle and she was probably happy that I had this safe outlet for my worries. It was like my first positive experience with a 'therapist'.

We spoke about everything. I saw her as a friend and it was very easy to trust her. There wasn't anything I couldn't say to her. I would tell her if I was feeling down and what had happened to me during the week. It was an opportunity to talk without feeling judged and without putting on an act.

I continued to go to Michelle's regularly for five years, until about the age of 14, and then intermittently until my late teenage years. When I was older, I helped Michelle with the school holiday art classes she would run for little kids. I'd pour the paints and make sure the kids were polite and cleaned up. It felt like it was my studio too. I got on so well with the children that some of the parents asked me to babysit. This helped with my confidence and self-esteem, making money and having my own responsibilities.

As I got older, I'd phone Michelle up when I felt like having an art session with her. I was being much more experimental by that stage, working on canvasses rather than paper, and spray painting. While it was never about producing great art, I did produce some beautiful work that gave me great pleasure. Sometimes I'd just phone for a chat or we'd go out for coffee. We are no longer teacher and student. We might have an art-making session together but it is as two good friends.

One of the early things I did with Michelle was to make a book. I wrote the story, illustrated it and then bound it. It was called *A Very Hateful Giant* and, as I wrote on the back cover: 'It's a story about a giant named Hateful. He is very unfriendly and lives on top of a very lovely town named Lovely Ville ...'

The story, written when I was almost 11, was an expression of my own emotional turmoil. Like the giant, I just wanted to turn off that angry switch but I had no control over what was happening to me. I didn't have the tools to express my emotions but that book articulated exactly how I was feeling.

You can find the whole book reproduced within Chapter 8.

6

Unable to Walk the Talk

I didn't have any say in my high school and, even if I had, I wouldn't have known what to say or where to go. I would have only wanted to join my friends at whatever school they were heading off to.

What I did know is that the school my parents wanted to send me to was highly regarded as one of the best schools in the area. I felt I owed it to my parents to attend. I never told them that I didn't want to go. I was definitely never happy about it, but I resigned myself to it and went.

It was a huge change for me, coming from a school where I had a lot of female friends to a place with no girls and no existing friends. Unlike my very small and relaxed public primary school, this was a much larger, very structured environment and there was a very strict uniform policy. Already aware that I would be anxious about the move, my parents had organised for a private orientation of the school and made sure that there would be support if I needed it.

They had presented the school as offering me a lot more opportunities than the local public high school so I felt that it was probably the right place for me to go, even if I didn't want to be there.

Going to an all-boys school was very hard for me. There was a big focus on group sport, which I didn't like. Even when I chose to do swimming, I had become very self-conscious of my body because I had become quite overweight. I'd hide myself in a rash vest, which would slow me down considerably in the water. The one activity I loved now became a huge burden.

Of course, the level of set schoolwork also stepped up and I found there was a lot of pressure – again applied by myself – to do well academically. In the past, it had been easy to achieve good results with a reasonable amount of work. I had come from a school where you had an hour of homework every week and I could get that all done. Now, I had been put in all the extension classes so my daily workload would be up to three hours a night. On top of this were the assignments that required weekend attention.

This was a major adjustment for me because my downtime is a big part of my life. I need the space and time to be alone and unwind. When I was young, I'd spend time with my grandparents or the dog. At home, I'd play Lego or watch whatever was on TV. There was no time for those distractions anymore. I definitely found a huge amount of pressure at high school and I didn't feel connected to anyone because I didn't know anyone.

I don't think I was at the top of the year but I was still doing very well, even in the extension classes. However, assignments would stress me out to the point where I put them off and pretend they didn't exist until the night before they were due. That was a big change for me, the student who always wanted to finish everything the moment he got it. I still did well in assignments but I couldn't compartmentalise – doing a little bit now and a little bit later. It was either you do it all now or you do it all later. I had been able to do it 'right now' when it was a minor piece of primary school homework, but that was no longer an option. The inability to break a big task into smaller, manageable units proved a big stumbling block for me. I guess it would be described as lacking organisational skills.

Still, I was very good at suppressing how I felt and distracting myself. I was so unhappy at that school for a number of reasons: being isolated from my social network, an all-boys school, the huge focus on sport and the huge amount of work and homework. No pressure was coming from anyone but myself. My parents weren't saying: 'Why aren't you doing well? Why aren't you doing this?' There was always encouragement, but I felt such a burden to succeed, as well as to stay at this school. I didn't want to let my parents down.

***

During one of the school holidays, mum took Nathan and me down to Adelaide to visit her younger brother, Marc. He was living in an apartment on the beach and, still single, had just started seeing Emma, a lovely woman who would soon become his wife.

It was a wonderful break from Sydney for me but, even so, I was sometimes feeling too miserable to join in on the family outings and would stay in the unit on my own.

That first visit was such a pleasure, that I returned on a number of occasions over the following three years, and always on my own. Generally, I'd stay for a couple of weeks at a time, fitting right into Marc's new family. I was part of the family and felt completely at home.

Emma had a son from a previous relationship who was just a toddler at the time he came into Marc's life. Though no blood relation, he was just like me and we got on very well. Emma is only 13 years older than me – closer in age to me than she is to my mum – so she and Marc didn't feel like parents. They were more like a fun auntie and uncle.

And we did have fun! We'd go swimming, or play putt-putt golf. We always laughed and I had such a nice time there. It was a real escape from my everyday life and its woes, and because I knew I wouldn't bump into anyone I knew, that also relaxed me. There would be no questions to answer about how I was getting along and why I wasn't at school.

Marc and Emma always offered to have me and I would often ask to go. During those few years when my frequent visits to Adelaide helped sustain me, Emma became pregnant with twins and I experienced the joy of watching their family grow.

***

I'm not sure if my parents knew how unhappy I was at my new private school. With my dad, I only ever said what he wanted to hear, never what I thought. I filtered everything I said to him. My mum was always more aware of what was going on with me so she probably knew that something was not right. I didn't know how to express myself and, I suppose, I didn't feel I had the right to speak up.

I was phenomenal at wearing the 'everything's fine' mask, not just with my dad, but with everyone – friends, teachers and family.

But what I couldn't do with words, my body did with actions. All those miserable feelings were determined to come out, and if I wouldn't give them a voice, they would make themselves known in other ways. Basically, my body turned against itself. I didn't want to go to school but felt I had to; my body became sick so that I wouldn't have to go.

I can say this now with the benefit of hindsight. At the time, I was no more aware of why I was becoming ill than my parents, teachers or doctors. That first year of high school began with what I thought was a cold and resulted in me losing my voice. I was physically unable to speak up about my feelings. How apt was that! But this inconvenience was to be replaced by a more serious affliction: I lost the ability to walk. First I could not speak out against school; then I could not make my way to school.

It was a gradual build up of pain in my knees. The pain kept getting worse and it coincided with the introduction of school sport and my parents having just purchased me a brand new pair of soccer boots. I really didn't want to play sport. Around this time, the school camp was taking place. All the boys in my year were heading off for the great outdoors and some male bonding. I had to go, but my legs were causing me such grief that I had to be excused from many of the activities and I really didn't participate fully in the exercise.

My parents hoped that being away from the classroom, enjoying the fresh air and camaraderie of the other students might see me return in improved health and mobility. Instead, the pain only increased to the point where I couldn't get myself to school without my mother accompanying me and supporting my not inconsiderable weight. In the end, she had to get me crutches. I was limping wherever I went.

We went to see a doctor and the eventual diagnosis was Osgood-Schlatter disease, an adolescent condition to do with bone growth, which happens to teenage boys in particular. I was told basically that my legs were growing faster than the muscles around them.

If you look Osgood-Schlatter disease up on the Internet you'll find that it is characterised by painful lumps just below the knee. In my case, I had the pain but no lumps. You'll also find that a risk factor is excess weight and, sure enough, I ticked that box. But the other risk factor of overzealous running and jumping was certainly not an issue for me.

My mother was trying to keep me at school again, for as long as possible, and making sure I didn't have an excuse not to go. When it had been the cough and sore throat earlier in the year and I'd tried to stay at home, she'd told me I could still go to school. And when I lost my voice, she reiterated that sentiment, saying that even if I couldn't talk, the teachers would be happy to see me there. She wouldn't accept any of my excuses.

My high school was on a hill and there were a lot of stairs that were impossible for me to negotiate in my debilitated state. Instead of going to my classrooms, which were an obstacle course away from the roadside entrance, I would go to the much more conveniently located library. I don't know how she managed to do it but my mum virtually had to drag me there, support my weight plus my excessively heavy bag of 10 plus kilos of books that had to be carried around. In the library, I'd sit all day and do my work. The teachers would come up and give me the work I had to do and I was excused from classes. In my little sanctuary, it was better than being in class. I was happy up there, and especially thrilled to be excused from sport as well. The school was certainly very accommodating, making sure that my immobility impinged as little as possible on my education.

However, one morning I woke up and my leg was excruciatingly painful. You could touch my leg as gently as you would touch a baby, and it felt like someone was hitting me with a hammer. I was simply unable to walk and the pain could no longer be ignored.

The increased severity of the pain resulted in a referral to the pain management team at a major Sydney hospital. They ran a series of tests including X-rays, MRIs – everything. They admitted me into the hospital and I remained there for six weeks.

A stream of specialists, including an occupational therapist, physiotherapist, pain management doctor and a psychologist were constantly visiting me. I had to learn to walk again.

As far as my parents knew, I had a real physical condition, not an emotional one, but as it progressed, they started to have their doubts. My mother spoke with her brother and confided her suspicions to him. He recommended she read a book, which she says was very helpful to her: *How to Stop Worrying and Start Living*, by Dale Carnegie. Written over half a century ago, it is probably one of the first 'self-help' books that have risen to international acclaim.

　　　　　　　　　　　　　　　　　　　　　　mum, i wish i was dead

What my mother gleaned from the book is that emotional pain can present itself in a physical way. My nanna had been pestering my mother to ask for brain scans, frightened that a neurological disorder might be behind my inability to walk, but my mother told her, 'I think this is an emotional problem we are dealing with'. The doctor had already spoken with my mother and said that he didn't think a brain scan was necessary.

At the time, I wasn't aware of any of this.

Apparently the hospital put me on a very mild antidepressant, which was used for amputees because the pain I was feeling was like a phantom pain. My parents were also called in to see the hospital psychiatrist.

My mother says that it was during my hospital stay that she changed her mindset and went against the advice of professionals whose focus was to get me back to school. 'We are not going to focus on getting Adam to school. We are going to focus on getting Adam well. Whatever that takes.'

After my release, I still had to visit the hospital six days a week for hydrotherapy. I also had to visit the psychologist twice a week, and then once a week after I'd returned to school. Eventually, I transitioned to seeing my own psychologist. The hospital had put me on cognitive behaviour therapy (CBT).

A simplified explanation of CBT is that it is about trying to think yourself out of a bad feeling if there is no rational explanation for it. So, for example, if you are anxious about going somewhere, you have to think why it is you are suffering from the anxiety, and if it is not a rational reason, then think yourself out of the anxiety.

A lot of the time we went over the same process again and again and it made me feel stupid. I'm a logical person and always have been, but this approach felt like I was being treated as if I were a young child. I didn't want to continue with it. I needed something different.

CBT does work for some people, and in retrospect I can say that it did help me with mild anxiety and taught me several tools I occasionally use today. However, I had deeper issues that it wasn't reaching.

***

As the year was drawing to a close, I dreaded the thought that I would be coming back to the school the following year. Things hadn't improved at all since those early days. Still, I didn't tell my parents. I had told the psychologist about my antipathy and it is possible that he shared that knowledge with them.

My mother came to realise that being at this school was no longer the best thing for me and had to back-peddle on the sales pitch she'd given me about it. She explained why she had presented my current school in a good light and why she now felt another school might be better for me. It wasn't a hard sell. I was more than happy to be farewelling my private boys' school and heading off to the local public high school where I would be reunited with many familiar faces.

I had only lasted at that private school for a year. With the promise of a change of school and a new start, things settled down again and the pain gradually disappeared.

It is only with hindsight I understood that the whole episode of not being able to walk was just a physical symptom of an emotional problem. I now realise that every physical ailment I've ever had, including severe bouts of constipation when I was younger, has been associated with an emotionally distressing situation. That was the first major one that hit me. I was very sick that year and those physical manifestations were definitely related to my inability to express verbally how unhappy I was. I didn't know how to get myself out of school so my mind attacked my body.

That whole year was horrible. It affected every area of my life. I didn't make any friends, just acquaintances. One of the few bright spots was my hospital stay when all my friends from primary school came to visit me. We were able to leave the hospital and we went to see a movie at the local cinema; I went in a wheelchair. That was nice, but it also reminded me of what I was missing and how happy I had been, so the experience was bittersweet.

I also enjoyed speaking openly with my psychologist. He was very comforting, and I remember feeling very good after every time we met. He never spoke of my condition as being a psychological one. I believed he was there to see if there were any problems at home. I may have told him I was unhappy at school and I think he passed that on.

With the promise of good things to come, I was getting excited about entering my second year of high school. Perhaps my life would be getting back on track.

mum, i wish i was dead

7

Adolescent Angst

After discussing other school options we looked at my local high school and decided to start there. I knew a lot of the kids there from primary school and some of those I knew but hadn't really been close to, soon became my best friends.

Almost from the moment I started in Year 8, everything changed and I was happy. A huge burden was removed from my shoulders and I loved being at school again. There were girls, a relaxed atmosphere and no sport. Not surprisingly, my health improved. Life was great again.

The school was split into two campuses. Plans for the future of the school involved selling off one site and using the funds to redevelop the other where, eventually, all classes would be consolidated.

But at the time I joined, the campus was pretty empty, with only Years 7 and 8 students housed there. The other Years, 9–12, were located at the other campus. Having come to it in Year 8, I was among the older kids there, which was a good feeling. I was more or less at the top of the pecking order and I fitted in well.

I wasn't overly popular. I didn't have lots of friends but I had a few close friends – and that was all I needed. I could keep up with the work and the teachers were good, so everything was going well. There were all the typical teenage issues of girls and school generally, but nothing too serious. Having said that, I did have a 'girlfriend' at the time and that ended disastrously.

Maybe missing that first year of high school and being cloistered away from girls for that period put me at a slight disadvantage. Early adolescence is a funny age, where you have to make the transition from mixing with girls comfortably as equals, to developing an interest in them as the other sex. I'd enjoyed the company of all my female classmates in primary school, but that year away from them may have hindered the transition into forming more intimate relationships, which is never easy in the best of circumstances.

I was such a serious and sensitive boy; I didn't understand all the game playing that goes on in early relationships. It seemed like it should be straightforward to me: you liked someone and you let them know so you could spend time with them. The intrigue of when and where to reveal your hand, to affect disinterest when you were keen were completely foreign and alien tactics to me.

However, at the age of 14, I didn't want to be the only guy who hadn't kissed a girl.

There was one girl who I liked very much, but I had no confidence to say or do anything with her. She lived on my walking route to school and some mornings we would walk to school together. I wanted to kiss her but I didn't dare try. Eventually the relationship developed and we would start to see each other outside of school times and speak on MSN all the time. We had mobile phones and we'd message each other so I burned through my credit in no time.

She had a lot of issues with her own family and we'd talk about it. No one would ever know about her problems from looking at her. She appeared remarkably together. I was a sympathetic ear, wanting to provide whatever support I could.

Our friendship progressed quite quickly, probably because of the kind of person I am, which is reasonably intense. And I do crave closeness from those I care about. We were always 'on' and 'off', and every time we were 'off' it would devastate me. We ended up dating for about six months, which felt like a lifetime at high school. As we shared a lot of classes together, it was quite involved when we were 'on' because we spent so much time in each other's company. This was definitely first love.

When we were messaging each other, she would always ask, 'what do you want to do with me?' And I'd always be the nice boy, saying that I didn't want to do anything until she was ready. And she always said, 'I just want you to tell me, I want to be with you'. I guess it was a bit of a tease on her part, and must have added some excitement to that dance around the issue that preoccupies young kids.

One day she messaged me with the same question, 'What do you want to do with me?' I was with my mates at the time and I shared the text with them. What was I meant to do with this continuous querying of my desires and intentions? It was the wrong place to be considering this question, with all those teenage boys pumped up on hormones and getting a vicarious thrill from my love life.

'Man up and tell her,' they said. Easy for them, as they weren't doing the deed themselves. However, there is a bravado in such groups that can lend you the bravery you need. Also, the distance of texting makes it much easier to speak your mind than to open up to someone in person.

So that afternoon, I finally did tell her what I wanted. It wasn't in any graphic detail, but I said, 'I want to sleep with you'. Pretty tame, really, and I didn't have any idea of what to do with her, even if her response was going to be positive.

The response I did receive was another text message a little time later saying, 'Call me.' I was still with my mates so I didn't call immediately. When I had a moment of privacy, I rang her number with some anticipation and excitement.

However, it wasn't my girlfriend who answered the phone. It was her step-dad, and he went off, abusing the hell out of me. Somehow he had seen my message saying that I wanted to sleep with his daughter and he'd been the one to lure me into making the phone call. He was screaming and seriously threatening me. It was certainly not what I was expecting to hear on the other end of the line and I was completely stunned.

At the time, I didn't realise what was going on. And then it hit me. It dawned on me that there was an adult who wanted to cause me harm and that, one way or another, my girlfriend and I had broken up.

At school I was threatened from going anywhere near her. We'd still speak on MSN occasionally but that confrontation ended our relationship. I felt threatened for my life, to the point that if we were seen speaking at school together, her mum would chase me and I had to run off. I'd be virtually in tears and have to call my mum to pick me up. I'd clearly made a reputation for myself, which was completely unwarranted. I was such a safe boy who hadn't lifted a finger, even in the face of much encouragement.

My mother had to phone the girl's parents to say that it was not okay to threaten kids. Yes, what I did was wrong, but their response was not right either. It was my first perceived love and that definitely did hurt. She was a very attractive girl and lots of guys flirted with her, which used to bother me.

There was some kind of game-playing going on, because on MSN she used to say that she still liked me and missed me, but then at school she completely ignored me. I am much more inclined to go cold turkey, so I backed off emotionally. I was burnt and didn't want to keep exposing myself to more disappointment.

But while I developed a protective coating by not allowing myself to get involved again, I did maintain contact, replying when she initiated a conversation online. I said to her, 'if you ever need something, just let me know'. If you love someone, you are there for them. I knew she had been through a lot and had her own traumas.

A month or two would pass without a word and I would have gotten her out of my system, then she'd send me a text message and reel me back in again. It would just be a message to say, 'I need you'. I could never say no, whether the love was there or not. Whenever I would agree to see her, it would bring back the feelings. She had an exquisite sense of timing, knowing exactly when she'd left the silence long enough and ran the risk of me breaking loose from her hold.

The summer holidays came and went with relative uneventfulness. I'd spent time with my friends but there was no love interest on the horizon. There was no summer romance. Nothing happened. I'm a guy who loves to love and I'm very passionate.

***

It was soon time to move from the small pond of the first campus and join the bulk of the school at the second where Years 9–12 congregated. Now I was among the very youngest on a big new campus.

It was the start of Year 9 and it wasn't just the school location that changed. I also moved out of home to my nanna and poppa's place. This

mum, i wish i was dead

was a comfortable, safe place for me and probably gave the family a bit of a breather too. Being out of each other's way would hopefully allow family interactions to improve, and it was my choice to go.

It is hard to remember the exact reason why I moved out. However, with hindsight it would have been a combination of things – the tension at home between my dad and me, as well as with my brother would have become too much. Then there was mum always asking if I was okay, which left me feeling hassled. All of these things were underpinned most likely by an unrecognised depressive episode.

Nonetheless, it wasn't a huge upheaval because my grandparents live only a short distance from our home, and I was used to spending a great deal of time with them throughout my childhood. Also, I was still seeing my family on a daily basis. I had the luxury of enjoying two addresses.

My dad would drop by every night to say hello. Sometimes I was with friends or just not interested and didn't see him, but my nanna would always let me know he'd come. We still had a strained relationship and I wasn't always keen to catch up with him. I had always felt like I had to become someone I wasn't to please him and I never felt comfortable just being me. He had such an easy-going relationship with Nathan and I could see he was proud of him. It wasn't the same with me. I felt I was a disappointment to him. It's hard to put my finger on any specific thing that was said or done – it was just how I felt.

Although we bonded over a few things, the main one was Lego. Men have to bond over something, so we were lucky there was that one thing we both loved. Most of our arguments centred around food because I was stacking on the weight. Though his motivation was to protect me, I was not mature enough to read it as anything other than disapproval for who I was.

Besides, I craved food. Some days I had an appetite that couldn't be satisfied. There was definitely a correlation between my binge eating and how bad my mood was. The food would give me a sense of goodness and I would feel better. When I was bad, all I wanted to eat was sweet things. I would consume an entire litre of icecream in one sitting. Anything high in fat and sugar, as well as extra large portions – that was for me. If there was food in the fridge, I ate it. I was on a search and devour mission.

Dad had a 'look' on his face whenever I wanted something when we were out or I was asking for an extra portion at the table. Whether he was aware of it or not, it was there and said more than any words could. Every time I saw that look I felt like he was asking 'Do you *really* need it?' That made me furious. I felt so patronised, and so I did most of my binge eating in secret. I'd also come to accept that I would be overweight forever and my ravenous eating for comfort would always be like this.

Fortunately, what had been the cause of the greatest friction between my father and me became the spur for the mending of our relationship: we started going to the gym together.

At the age of 14 when everyone becomes painfully conscious of their appearance I was still overweight. Instead of focusing on my eating, which was having negative repercussions, my dad suggested that exercise might be the way for me to shed some kilos. Suddenly, I had an activity to throw myself into and a buddy with whom to do it – my dad.

At the start, dad would pick me up from my grandparents' place a couple of afternoons a week and we'd go to the sports complex on the fringe of Sydney's CBD. As time progressed, we'd go more frequently and sometimes even on the weekend. As well as using the gym, we'd have some personal training sessions. There was a female trainer who managed the gym who was there most of the time. She continuously gave me encouragement and support. It was nice being acknowledged by a girl.

After being dogged by my weight for the past few years, I wanted to get fit and healthy. I had associated exercise with playing sport, which I didn't like, so the gym was a saving grace for me and I developed my love of gym workouts here. There was no competition and you got to work at your own pace. What's more, I was good at it and I thrived in this environment.

My dad also enjoyed seeing me exercising and having fun. The experience created the building blocks for our relationship. It was at the gym that we took the first steps in developing our positive father-son relationship. In fact, things were going so well that I decided to move back home. The kilos were also coming off and I was looking good and feeling good. Dad now had a new 'look' on his face – he didn't need to say anything, but I could see he was proud of me.

Out of the blue, my ex-girlfriend messaged me, asking if I wanted to walk to school with her the next day. Even though we had changed campuses, we both still lived in walking distance to school. I ignored the message, and when I arrived at school the next day, she wasn't there. That got me worried. She only messaged me if she needed something so I wondered if something bad had happened to her. And hadn't I told her some months before that if she ever needed to talk, I would be there for her? The absence of contact had led me to believe that she had moved on and had no need for my friendship or counsel.

When I got home that evening, I went straight on MSN and she was on there, too. I asked what her message the previous day was about. 'Why weren't you at school?'

She said, 'I wanted to apologise and give you something to make up for everything I put you through.'

So I said, 'Okay, let's meet up tomorrow and walk to school.'

When we started walking, it was like being transported back to the best time of our friendship. We were talking and laughing, until I got around to asking her what she had wanted to talk about. All of a sudden, her mood changed. She acted as if nothing had happened. It was really strange and upsetting. I became very emotional and said, 'This is ridiculous'. I have always hated being lied to.

As she walked off and left me behind, all the feelings came rushing back. We hadn't really addressed anything. That was that. I'd been duped again. She'd reeled me back in, once more, but this was the last time. I got over that experience much quicker than the times before. I became resigned to how the relationship was going to run. We did become some sort of friends, but the heat and confusion dissipated.

That was at the start of Year 9 and, in spite of the hiccup, it was a great year. I didn't have a girlfriend but I was with friends. We'd go to each other's houses and we'd sneak alcohol, or go to the park and socialise around bonfires. We were just being teenagers and pushing boundaries. I was more the one that tagged along than the person who came up with the ideas of mischief or planned our social activities.

I was never in any particular group. The lines were much more fluid for me. I don't know how 10 people can all get along and like each other equally.

I was always good friends with one or two people in each group, girls as well. So I did have a lot of friends who had allegiances to their groups, but I'd spend time with them on their own, occasionally getting to know them very well. That was my friendship dynamic at school.

Academically, things were going along well, too. In fact, classes were easy for me and I'd reached the point where I was getting a little bored in class and then I'd be ticked off by the teacher for not paying attention. That year, my life was back on track: I'd lost weight, had friends and I was happy. Nothing bad had happened.

As school ended for the year in December, I celebrated my 15th birthday. The summer holidays were around the corner. Our family had started to go on holidays over the New Year period because they didn't want us in Sydney getting caught up in the drama of New Year's Eve celebrations.

I loved family holidays, but for some reason I didn't want to join this trip. I fundamentally refused to go. Whether it was fear of missing out on something happening in Sydney, or wanting to be with my friends, I did *not* want to go on the holiday.

The holiday was planned for a resort in the US. It would have been a fantastic treat, so my parents must have puzzled over why I was so determined to avoid it. I think that's when alarm bells started ringing for my mum. I'd been getting agitated and moody. Anytime she'd ask me something, I'd snap at her, saying, you have no idea! I'd push back.

In the end, there was nothing for them to do but go on holiday and leave me behind. They all went away but I stayed with my grandparents down the road. I'd sleep at their place and come back to the house during the day.

8

It Has a Name: Depression

My parents were only gone for a few weeks, and since I loved staying with my grandparents who always spoilt me rotten, that was no hardship.

My parents came back and the school year started. But almost as soon as the holidays had ended, it became clear that I was descending into another bad space. Mum knew something wasn't right, I knew something wasn't right, but I still had no idea how to express it.

I don't recall being taught this at home, but in society males seem to be taught to suppress their feelings, to toughen up. If you do feel bad, you're taught to think positively, or forget it because tomorrow is another day. That's all well and good generally, if you have a bad moment or two. For me, the issue was that the next day was never any better. The next day was the same, if not worse. Consecutive bad days, without a break from these debilitating thoughts and feelings, take a significant toll, both physically and emotionally.

Because my closest family relationship was with my mum, she copped the worst of it. I guess it is a sign of how secure I felt with mum that I could save my worst outbursts for her, although that would have been cold comfort for her to know. I definitely took for granted that my family, and mum in particular, would always be there for me, no matter how poorly I behaved.

Any question directed to me, even an innocuous enquiry about how I was going or what I was doing, would send me right off. It sounds crazy, but I felt judged or ridiculed.

Most nights of the week, mum, dad, Nathan and I would sit down for dinner and talk. One night, as we were sitting at the table eating our meal, something was said that annoyed me. It can't have been so significant because I don't even remember what the comment was. Whether it was about school, food, girls, my weight or whatever else may have triggered me, I am not entirely sure. None the less, something was said that sent me over the edge.

Whatever it was, I lost it. I snapped. Standing up and slamming my fists on the table, I called them fucking idiots and said, 'I'm done with all your shit; I'm leaving'. I was very angry and I swore as I stormed to my room, wedging something into the door to keep them out.

I'd always had my moments but I'd never acted like this before. My parents didn't try to stop me because I was a big child and they couldn't restrain me. They were also probably shocked by the outburst and unsure of what to do. I'm sure they knocked on my door as they went to bed. However, I am unsure of my response.

Once I knew everyone had gone to sleep, I left. I attempted to sneak out of the house without anyone knowing. I didn't want to be in this home anymore.

It was coming into autumn so the night was chilly. Our house is up near the sea and there is a long strip of grass close to the cliffs where it is pleasant to take in the view during the daytime. Now it was dark and freezing cold, and I was out there alone. I settled down on the gym equipment at the local reserve and looked up at the stars.

Although it felt like time had stopped, I mustn't have been out there for too long as my parents heard the front door and were obviously worried and had come looking for me. Luckily I wasn't as quiet leaving as I had thought. They found me lying in silence. Dad was there but I don't recall him saying anything. I don't know what could have even been said. Mum was talking frantically, trying to find out what was happening to me. I wasn't responding at all, only tears were rolling down my cheeks. Eventually, I poured out my heart. I wasn't happy. I wanted to die. I didn't know why or what to do. Saying this out loud made me finally realise something was very wrong.

When they got me back home, my mother said, 'This is beyond me. I don't know what to do about your situation. I'm not skilled.' She said she would take me to see the GP in the morning, but that even she may not be able to help me either and she may refer me onto someone else. We still didn't know what we were dealing with. We still didn't know it was depression.

Mum thought it would be best to go to our local doctor rather than a hospital because she felt that if we sought private healthcare, the response would be much quicker and we would have more control. She didn't want me sitting around a waiting room in the state I was in.

When we went to the GP the next day it was very clear I needed to go on medication. I was incredibly sad and I didn't want to live. Because I was under 16, the doctor couldn't prescribe anything for me on the spot. She needed to refer me to a psychiatrist – and quickly.

The GP went onto a website that was supposed to provide 24-hour assistance to doctors, only to be asked to leave her number with the promise that they would get back to her. That wasn't good enough. I needed to get to a psychiatrist as soon as possible.

The doctor and my mother started calling around to find a colleague or friend who could organise an emergency appointment. Even the two receptionists at the practice were so concerned that they rallied around to find someone for me. One of the women said she knew a psychiatrist who was very good and she was able to get us in to see him that afternoon.

On the way over, my mum tried to prepare me: 'Adam, you need help now. You may or may not like this psychiatrist. If you don't like him, we will change. But you need help now.' I agreed with her. I was feeling so desperate and wanted someone to help me get better.

The reason my mum was anxious about me getting on with the psychiatrist was because I had a bad experience with one at the age of 10. I hated it. That particular time we'd been as a family to the psychiatrist and I really didn't want to go. I'd been against the idea from the start. I sat there slumped down in the chair with my hoodie over my head, refusing to say a word. I was very resistant to the whole idea, maybe because I didn't want the whole family there. My brother, Nathan, on the other hand, loved it. Even though we were there because of my issues, it was the first time that someone wanted to hear from him and he was gearing up for the attentive audience.

Even though we hadn't been able to check around for recommendations and had to be grateful that any specialist could see me at such short notice,

I was very lucky. I liked this psychiatrist from the start, and he turned out to be amazing. I've been with him ever since.

He never made me feel rushed. With other doctors and counsellors, they are always watching the clock. He never makes you feel like you are a distraction and that he has better things to get on with. Even to this day, if anything goes wrong with me, I can send him an email and he'll respond quickly. Having spoken to other people about doctors they've seen, I know how fortunate I was to find a good one first time.

I was also able to be very open with him, and tell him how miserable and sad I'd been. My mother was present at the first session. Whenever professionals have asked me if I wanted my mother with me, I have always said 'Yes'. I want my parents to be as completely involved as possible. I know how much my mum worries and I didn't know how to deal with this on my own. I didn't want her to feel excluded and I knew I had a better chance of getting well with her support. She played no part in causing my unhappiness but she was suffering with me and had a right to be freed of my misery too.

I was diagnosed as being depressed. It was really the first time that my years of unhappiness had been given a name. We knew that I was suffering emotionally. Even my mum had figured that my period of not being able to walk had been triggered by something in my mind, but depression was not a condition she was familiar with. We didn't know anyone with depression or anyone who had gone through a depressive phase. It never occurred to my mum that this is what I had. How could I be depressed when I lived in a loving, stable family and appeared to have everything a child could want?

Just as the word 'depression' had never been used, neither had the word 'suicidal'. Even though I didn't want to live, I never associated these thoughts as being suicidal thoughts, and clearly they were.

Strangely, it was comforting to have a name for the way I felt. It's terrible when you are suffering from something that feels so innately wrong, but no one acknowledges it. No one knows what it is, no one sees it, there's no scan for it, there's nothing to determine what it is. Yet here is a doctor, an obvious professional in his field, saying, 'This is what you have, this is what it means, and these are the treatment options'.

You go, 'Okay, it's something that can be treated. It's not just me. It's not my fault; it's not something I did or that someone else did.' The diagnosis alleviated some of the burden because I had no idea why I was feeling this way. The suggestion was made that it was a chemical imbalance, and at last that was something I could grapple with. Not just a name but an explanation as well. It was a huge relief.

This psychiatrist asked all the right questions and he explained what was going on. The acknowledgement of mental illness in adolescents is relatively new. The idea has been around for perhaps 20 years. Most of these emotional upsets were attributed to growing up: 'just a stage he's going through'.

Now, instead of having the label 'teenage angst', my problems were given a different label. That didn't bother me. People complain about labelling and it turns them off. 'So and so is depressed; another person is bipolar; someone else has ADD.' But the labels are about the diseases, not the person, and it's important to name them and speak about them.

If someone has cancer, you don't know them as 'the person who has cancer'. We still know them as 'them', and it's just that they're suffering from cancer. People suffer from depression and they suffer from bipolar. It doesn't make them who they are.

That's something even I learned to understand all through my recovery. The depression didn't make me, 'me'. It was just another event in my life that would be part of moulding me for the future.

Just because you have one of these diseases doesn't make it you. There is a great fear that, once you get diagnosed with depression, you are labelled or stigmatised for life. It's as if the label makes it true and permanent, and that's worse for some people. They have to realise that this diagnosis doesn't change who they are, it just allows them to have a thing that they can name and treat. Not naming it doesn't make it go away. It will always be there regardless of you acknowledging it. However, once you know what you have, you know how to fight it.

While it was good to feel that my problems were now going to be addressed, I also felt very alone. If people don't like talking about mental health in adults, it is even more rarely discussed in adolescents. Was I the only teenager out there with this disease? I'd been happy to be ahead of my peers at schoolwork, but I didn't want to claim any victory for achieving an adult disorder at such a young age. No prizes there.

Because I hadn't heard about depression, there was a nagging thought at the back of my mind: is the doctor just saying this to make me feel better? Was it his way of being sympathetic, reassuring me that I wasn't the only one and there are a lot of people who have it? I certainly hadn't met anyone else like that. Or should I say, like me. I had no idea.

If depression occurs so frequently, why hadn't I seen it before? Why didn't people talk about it? I guess that was the naivety of the 15-year-old I was. Those were the thoughts playing around in my head: that there was this huge, secret world of depression that everyone had been complicit in keeping silent about, or there weren't many people suffering with this problem and I was really the odd one out, but being made to feel as if I was one of many and not so strange.

Only later did I understand the stigma surrounding depression.

My condition was described as acute, and I needed to be put on medication immediately. Acute means that you not only have suicidal thoughts but that you will act on them, and I didn't feel I could stop myself from acting out my thoughts. I wasn't afraid of dying. The fear is about continuing to live as you are. That's what drives you to it. It feels like the only way to get the misery to stop is to kill yourself.

Outsiders often believe that suicide is a selfish act, claiming that those who succumb are only thinking about themselves, not how their actions will devastate their friends, family and loved ones. But when you are depressed, your capacity to be rational is undermined.

No matter how much my mother told me she loved me, a lot of the time I thought she was only saying it because she had to; a line mothers are expected to take. I didn't actually believe her. My understanding of reality was seriously distorted.

You also desperately want to end your pain. You've tried everything else without relief. And when you reach that stage where suicide seems like the only option, it's not as if you haven't contemplated it before. In fact, the reason you haven't acted for so long is because you *do* worry about the hurt you will cause others. You don't just wake up one morning and think, 'I'll do it!' You have been suffering for a prolonged period of time, and you have seen the pain your suffering has caused others. I saw the damage I didn't mean to do, but had: the disruption to our usual family life; the endless appointments

mum, i wish i was dead

with doctors; the pain on my mother's face as I'd talked about my desperation and wish to end it all.

Sometimes, you even think you will be doing others a favour. Though I knew they would be hurt initially, I thought I'd be reducing their pain in the long term. They could stop worrying about me. Instead of anguishing when they went to bed at night whether I'd be alive in the morning, they'd know 'it' had been done. That would stop the misery for all of us.

I'd never been at this point before that night in the park. I'd definitely imagined what it would be like for me not to be here. When a car would drive across the road, I used to think, 'What if I step in front of it?' Or I'd stand at the top of the stairs and imagine myself lying at the bottom and think, 'Would that be an easier way to end it?' But previously I had only toyed with these ideas. Now I was serious about them.

The psychiatrist started me on a drug and arranged another appointment again in a week to see how I responded. In the meantime, I was closely monitored. That was the beginning of 15 months of trialling different medications, none of which were ideal.

I realised that I'd been unhappy for a few months. That's why I didn't go on the big family holiday. There was no trigger to it, but every day I'd been getting worse. I was frustrated and angry, and I was constantly wearing the mask in public to pretend everything was good. I'd been feeling all this stuff for months before. There's only so long you can wear that mask. It is indescribably draining, both physically and emotionally, to have a mask on pretending to the world that you are okay, when you are being crushed inside.

At the beginning, you put on the mask to deny to yourself how awful you are. If you put on a positive face, you reason, then everything will be alright. Later you wear the mask to stop others seeing your true self and to protect them from how hateful you feel yourself to be. I wanted school friends to like me and include me in their activities, not shun me because I was severely depressed. And I didn't want to horrify the people I loved.

I was so good at wearing this mask that over the years, both before and after my diagnosis with depression, parents in our circle of friends would come up to my mum and dad and say something along the lines of, 'Adam is fine. He is smiling, laughing and playing.' The people who had regularly been in my life since birth couldn't see anything wrong with me. They couldn't understand how I could be depressed, how I could be allowed to miss school. 'Adam seems normal. He is good and well behaved. Nothing is wrong.'

I wasn't okay; the mask I wore allowed me to seem 'normal' and happy. A smile and good behaviour doesn't mean things are fine. It didn't mean things weren't wrong. I was always depressed. My behaviour changed with how full my 'volcano' was. The mask drained what little energy I had and when I had nothing left, when my volcano was full, the mask came off. I always knew when I was getting to my limits and had to be removed from public and returned home where I could let my true self come out.

At my Year 6 farewell, my parents had to be called to pick me up. At every birthday party, New Year's Eve, at any celebration where I was usually surrounded by my closest friends and family, I had to leave early. I never wanted anyone to experience how bad I actually was. I didn't want to be judged any more than I already felt judged, and I didn't want to embarrass my family. Once I let the dark emotions out, allowed the volcano to explode, I could put the mask back on. I could appear 'normal' and well behaved. I could put on the smile and act how society expected. That is what it always was, an act.

I didn't believe I was a person anymore. There was this diseased thing, this monster, inside me. So I tried to wear the mask of how I remembered myself being, of how I ought to be. But you can only wear it for so long before you need to go to your own space and let the monster out.

With no idea about who to tell or what to say, there was something beyond my comprehension going on inside me. It was like a volcano bubbling away, waiting to erupt. There was no safety valve to release the pressure.

***

mum, i wish i was dead

Date: 2 May 2006 (aged 15 years)

From: Adam
To: Anne (mum)

If you where wondering this is how I feel (sorry about the spelling) ...

I hate my life right now like I cant stand how it is tonight I wanted to throw my self down the stairs just to avoid another day my life repeats it self over and over I hate it I don't want to go on and if I do I am extremely worried that dangerous things will happen to my self or others I will one day go to far and hurt myself terribly and if its not me it will be someone else if they piss me off that much I will hurt them too much I don't enjoy any day no matter what I do and now there is school I don't wake up and feel happy I wake up and wish I never did friends I thought I had I don't and impressions I got form people I was wrong I am continuously being hurt by people over and over it doesn't stop I feel like shit I just want to leave everything I don't care if I die or I leave or everything just stops I just cant do this any more its been like this for six years and it shits me that nothing has changed even though I have and I hate it I cry my self to sleep and everything for me is an effort I get so frustrated doing things because I am always having to work for myself I cant just ever be happy I have to work for it and no matter how hard I work or how hard I try I am still in the same position as before and every time I think its all going to be ok it isn't and everything fucks up again I am so

unhappy I cant sleep because I roll around and yes
I even tried reading but no it still did not work
I am so sick of how everything is in a cycle and a
bad cycle nothing can be good for me I want to wake
up happy I want to smile because I feel like smiling
not because I feel I have to I want to just enjoy my
life and who I am and what I am doing and who I am
with I don't and I haven't I put on this fake smile
and laugh and yes everything is good I cant take it I
don't want to take it anymore I cry all I do is cry I
have nothing else exercise only subsides the problems
but they r all still there I still cry after gym and
when I am with someone I have to hold it back I feel
like crying because I feel my life is so hard and yes
I am sure people go through it but know one does at
my age since I was ten it has been bad and continues
to get worse I just want to fit in I want to be happy
instead of sad I want to wake up and not feel worried
about what will happen during that day and be able
to fall asleep at night with out tears I don't look
forward to anything I have no inspiration even when
we were going to the sea food restaurant I wasn't
even looking forward to it I couldn't have even cared
less what happened and at art nothing comes I cant do
anything anymore sometimes I just wish I get hit by
a car or that a terrorist blows a car up into me or a
bus while I am on it or anything I just hate it all
and I have for a long time I am emotionally drained
I am still here but I feel like I am not here my body
is but my mind is dead I am not wanting my life I
know it is only going to get worse it always does I no
longer know how I am going to deal with what I can do
but the only thing I do know is that I can no longer
continue like this I decided to write it out because
I think this every night and I cant sleep so here it

mum, i wish i was dead

is its 1:22 am and I probably wont be asleep until 2 or 3 am which sucks because all I want is my sleep and that's something I cant get at night which leaves me physically exhausted as well as emotionally so I have no idea of what to do but that is basically how I feel at this very moment and how I have been feeling for a long time and most likely will continue to feel this way for unfortunately a very long time so now you have it in writing ...

Date: Monday, 22 May 2006

From: Adam
To: Hugh (my psychiatrist)

hi hugh its adam

i am using my mums email just to let you know how things are going with me.

um things have not been good at all most nights i have terrible lows and my sleeping well i still find it very hard to fall asleep, but once I'm asleep i have not woken up again like i did last week but i have felt very low and have wanted to throw myself down the stairs several times

i have silently cried almost every night and everything feels so hopeless and I'm still in a down not really caring about anything mood and I'm not sure really what to do

i am more sad than angry but at times i get angry
i get very frustrated quite quickly with things i
should and I'm over reacting and feel that i am
paranoid when consciously i know i shouldn't be but
i feel that way regardless of what I'm consciously
telling myself I'm also way over sensitive to things
that shouldn't even matter.

but yeh anyway i think that sums it all up really so
yeh just letting you know.

Date: Monday, 22 May 2006

From: Hugh
To: Adam

Hi Adam

Thanks for letting me know – hang in there with the
medication until I see you on Wednesday. I will talk
with you more about difficulty getting to sleep and
have a look at some strategies to help.

Hang in there Adam
HUGH

mum, i wish i was dead

Date: Friday, 9 June 2006

From: Anne
To: Tony (dad)

Hugh tried to contact me this morning to discuss a
plan of action for Adam after he had spoken with the
psychologist. When I rang back, he was busy.

In the meantime ...

On the way home from art this afternoon Adam told me
how sad he was, how he would prefer to be dead than
alive, that he has no control over anything and that
nothing works anymore. When we got home he slammed the
doors, went to his room, banged around a bit and threw
out the punching bag. I left him for a while and then
went up to him.

He was crouched on the floor sobbing. We both had a
cry and sat there for a while and then spoke a bit.
He doesn't want to go to hospital and is finding
everything so hard. He just can't do it anymore. We
knew his tutor was about to arrive and spoke to him
about doing his class with her and I said 'I don't
care if you only do crosswords' – it is all just too
hard.

I went downstairs to let his tutor in and speak with
her and apologise for not having the class today. As
she left, Hugh phoned.

I was on the phone for at least 30 mins with Hugh. Hugh asked a lot of questions and discussed a few things. He asked how I felt Adam had been doing over the past 4 weeks as his psychologist is very concerned about Adam also. As I felt Adam was getting worse we formulated a plan of action. The plan of action was to touch base with Sydney Children's Hospital. The belief is that Adam may need to be admitted tonight or over the weekend. I said to Hugh that I was very concerned about doing this as I didn't believe the support would be there over the weekend and he would be better at home as long as I could keep a close watch on him. At this point in time I wouldn't leave Adam unattended.

We are at a crisis point with Adam and I don't know which way things will go. It seems everyone is very concerned for his safety.

Anne

9

Struggling with Depression

The depression was so debilitating that I was unable to attend school for most of the next two years. Things had started to unravel from Year 10, even though the school was very supportive, having meetings with my family and making allowances for me. For example, I could go in late if I was on a new medication, and if I was feeling stressed or upset, I could leave the classroom and there was a safe place at school for me. I was trying to get back to school and the administration was doing what it could to make my return as smooth as possible.

One glitch came early in Year 10 when I was told that I wouldn't get my School Certificate because of my absences. It sent me into a complete spin. My education meant so much to me and my sense of worth was very much based on being a high achieving student. When I went home in distress and told my mother about this threat, she got straight on to the school. She spoke with the Deputy Principal at the time and said, 'Have you talked to Adam's Year adviser because she is very aware of what is going on? Maybe I should make an appointment to come in and see you.'

There was no sympathetic response from the Deputy. She was so aggressive that my mum said she needed to talk with her one-on-one. My mum also said, 'I think you have no understanding or idea about depression.' The Deputy replied, 'In fact I do. I had a son who was bipolar, schizophrenic and he committed suicide. So I know.'

My mum was bewildered as to why she was treating us like this. Luckily that woman left the school shortly afterwards.

In the hope of making the school more empathetic about my situation, my mother prepared a letter, briefing my teachers about what was happening with me and she went in and read it aloud to them. She has been very brave, on my behalf, and will do anything to smooth the way for me. She's also a strong believer in open communications, and I think that's one of the important lessons I've learned from her.

Mum's background help played a crucial role in my recovery and survival at the time. Here is the letter she read at school to the new Deputy Principal, my year co-ordinator and my other teachers who were able to attend:

Thank you for coming to this meeting today. I have put together this information to give you a better understanding of Adam and his needs.

When Adam was in year 5 (age 10) we first encountered issues with school refusal. At that time, Adam saw a psychologist and her main focus was to get Adam back to school. Over a period of time we achieved this.

In year 7 (age 12) Adam spent six weeks in hospital as he was unable to walk. Adam was under a team of professionals including a psychologist, physiotherapist, psychiatrist, pain specialist and occupational therapist. Once again, the main focus was getting Adam back to school.

In May this year, Adam lapsed into a deep depression with suicidal thoughts. We immediately sought professional help and since then Adam has been seeing both a psychologist and psychiatrist. The initial medication Adam was put on made Adam's condition worse and after a couple of weeks, this was changed. In the past few weeks, Adam has been put on medication for treatment of bipolar/manic depression. During the adjustment time of the medication, Adam no longer felt safe

mum, i wish i was dead

for himself and was concerned about the safety of others. We admitted Adam to hospital where he stayed for two nights.

Adam has not simply chosen not to be at school. He was deeply depressed, has had suicidal ideologies, has had his medication changed a few times as it wasn't working as hoped, learned he may have a chronic illness which is not well received or understood by the general public, dealt with me having a hysterectomy and has been hospitalised ... it is a lot for anyone to deal with in a 16-week period and he is only 15 years old.

Adam is now feeling well enough to return to school. In returning to school Adam has had to cope with his peers asking questions, adjust to a new campus, try and fit back into the classroom environment and deal with the work he has missed. All of this takes a lot of energy out of him. He hasn't used his brain, nor been so active for such a long time. The analogy we use to help Adam is that it is like when someone has broken a leg and the muscle withers. Once the plaster is off, it takes time and effort to get the leg working as it should and sometimes it is very painful and tiring doing the exercise required to get the muscles doing what they should. It is like this for Adam except that there is no visible physical injury.

After being back at school for only two days, he was told he probably won't get his School Certificate and had an altercation with a teacher. Yet despite these setbacks, Adam still came to school the next day. We admire Adam's strength in doing this.

I met many of you at the recent parent/teacher interviews and according to Adam, most of you have been very supportive of him. We thank you for this.

Tony and I believe Adam's health and wellbeing is of the utmost importance. We believe it is important for Adam to attend school regularly for both educational and social reasons. More importantly though is Adam's desire to complete his HSC and go on to tertiary education.

Those of you who have taught Adam in the past know he is a bright student who works independently and generally gets all work in by the due date. Hopefully with your patience and support, Adam will return to this within a short period of time.

In recent days, there has been a lot of focus or importance placed on Adam getting his School Certificate. Putting Adam under undue stress about getting his School Certificate will only exacerbate his problems at this time. Adam is not able to cope with the thought of repeating. Adam would see this as a punishment for something that is not in his control. In many ways he is more mature than his peers and as seen by his past results, he is bright enough to be pushed through. We will support Adam if private tuition is required to bring him up to date in subjects.

Our understanding of mental health issues and medication is that it is very difficult to diagnose adolescents. Finding a treatment that works is also trial and error. What works for one person may not work for another. We are still in the process of learning what will be best for Adam.

We believe it is important to remember that Adam is only 15 years old and is trying to deal with all of this the best he can.

Adam will continue to see his psychiatrist and psychologist who will work through issues with Adam as they arise.

Reasonable expectations:

- Adam attends school most days

- Adam may require time off to attend appointments with either his psychologist or psychiatrist. All effort will be made to ensure

mum, i wish i was dead

minimal disruption to school attendance. Adam's general appointment with his psychologist is on a Tuesday afternoon at 2:30pm. No other time is available. This may not be weekly.

- Adam is polite and respectful to teachers. If there is an issue, an appropriate time and place will be arranged to meet with the teacher and year adviser/school counsellor. If necessary, parents to be advised.

- Initially, homework and assignments may not be attempted.

- Adam to discuss with teachers issues relating to due dates of work set.

- Year Adviser to be advised of any changes to Adam's routine which would affect school.

- Teachers to notify parents of any concerns in relation to Adam

Adam, his psychiatrist and psychologist have read this. The only additional thought was from his psychologist who suggested a mentor at school for Adam. The reason is that if Adam has issues with a few subjects/teachers at one time, he would be able to go to one person rather than having to deal with several people. The person would also be a point of contact within the school if Adam feels the need to talk to someone about school related issues.

***

Although most of the teachers were extremely understanding, there were a few who definitely were not. One wrote an email to my mother saying, 'Adam didn't come to my class, yet I saw him in the playground and he was happy.' The teacher's response showed a complete lack of understanding about depression.

Parents will often complain that they can't get their kids to school yet the kids are up late at night, talking to their friends on Facebook. They just don't get that the most important thing for adolescents is to appear 'normal' with their peers. It's all part of the mask we struggle to put on when things go wrong. We want to fit in and that takes a lot of energy. It was more important for me to be mucking around with my friends like everything was fine than to sit through a lesson. I only had so much energy …

There were three incidents with teachers that I remember really setting me off. One was a teacher who directed a comment to me in front of the class. It was something along the lines of, 'Just because you have depression, that's no excuse. You still have to get your work done.' I just got up and left, heading straight to the First Aid room, which was my safe place. The mothers working in the office were very supportive and would all come in to see that I was okay and call my mum to let her know.

There was another incident with a different teacher and again I stormed out. Both of these teachers later apologised to me, and both ended up having their own anxiety and depression-related issues.

The other incident was with a teacher who I had asked to explain something I'd missed because of an absence. He wasn't very keen to go over it, implying it was my fault. This time I was furious and I left the room, pacing up and down the hall. I was so angry that I punched my fist through a door. I had to do it or I would have exploded.

The teacher walked out into the hall and I stopped and looked at him. He said, 'What did you do that for? What did the door ever do to you?'

I responded with, 'Would you prefer that to have been your face?'

A teacher came out from another classroom and diffused the situation. He said everything was alright. After that I went again to the First Aid room.

All my teachers knew what I was going through and, to be fair, most were terrific.

It's interesting that the teachers who had their own emotional problems or had first-hand experience of depression were the least sympathetic. Maybe they were resentful that I had been shown a lot of support and given a great deal of latitude while they had had to battle along on their own.

Ultimately, I was unable to spend much time at school. It just became too hard for me to go. I couldn't face it. It was very draining for my mother to have me around the house every day. At one stage, my nanna was also unwell, so mum was juggling the two of us. She says that the emotional strain for her came with seeing her child in pain, and not knowing what was going on. She also had Nathan's welfare to look after, a husband, a home to tend and a part-time job.

On top of that, not long after I started taking medication, mum had to have a hysterectomy and she was organising a family celebration for 200 people. So she had preparations to make and a celebration to organise. It was a very challenging time for mum.

She didn't like the idea of leaving me at home by myself, especially when I was bad, so if she couldn't be there, nanna would come over to keep me company. Later on when I was stronger and felt I could be on my own, I'd say, 'Mum, I'm fine. You can go out somewhere and leave me.' She had to learn to trust me, that I would let her know if I wasn't safe on my own. Although she now tells me that even once she had agreed to go out, she would ring nanna and get her to call me up. When I picked up the phone, nanna would say with apparent innocence, 'Oh, is mum at home?' It was mum's way of checking up on me without having to ring when she left the house to keep tabs on me.

My mum also tried to get me out of the house, finding an excuse to go out and have lunch at a café most days so I wouldn't stay stuck indoors and there would be a sense of purpose to my day. We'd go to the same comfortable, familiar coffee shop and we'd order the same food every day: chicken salad. We'd just duck down the road and be out for an hour. It was very simple and easy. It was probably my mother's way of freeing herself from the home, too, because while I stayed at home, she felt she needed to be there. Most of her energies and schedules were directed around me. During that time, there'd be days where if she only managed to get a load of washing on the line, she said she'd had a good day.

When I was at home I used to distract myself a lot with computer games. I couldn't sit with my own thoughts because they were too rapid and too morbid. My computer strategy games would provide an immersion for me and I would play them for hours. It would force my mind not to think. It would quiet the background noise.

There was also much watching of day-time TV with Oprah and Dr Phil. Oprah was on in the middle of the day and that show gave me hope when I was really bad. There were all these personal stories of tragedy, such as people living through floods or some other disaster. Although the stories made me sad, it was a 'happy sad'. There were people out there who cared enough about the plight of others to give and who would go out of their way to help. If those people could get through the horrific event that had befallen them, then I could get through my problems. That gave me a lot of hope.

mum, i wish i was dead

10

No Magic Pills

I couldn't sleep.

I avoided falling asleep because if I stopped having distractions, my mind would race a million miles. I was fearful of just lying quietly and allowing my mind to focus on my thoughts, so I had to wait until I was physically exhausted to go to sleep. That could be at three in the morning, and then I might not wake for another 12 hours. To be honest, I was fearful it would just be another day like the last and I didn't want that.

Staying awake watching television into the early hours, I saw a lot of silly late night advertisements. One night, an ad really spoke to me. Are you feeling x, y, z?, it asked. Then maybe you are bipolar. That just made me click. They were talking about all my symptoms. I went to the computer and started Googling, and thinking, 'this is me'. These words are describing how I am feeling.

The next time I saw my psychiatrist I suggested that this might be my problem, and we started introducing the mood stabiliser medications to the anti-depressants we'd been trialling. Sometimes these drugs work better together, and other times they work better when they are given separately. There didn't seem to have been much research on these medications in adolescents, so it was trial and error.

All I can say from my experience is that nothing worked for me. Almost everything I tried had terrible side effects, and the process of testing each drug regime took so much time. You have to allow so many weeks for the medication to build up in your system. Then you have to wait another few weeks to see if it works. And when it doesn't have the desired effect, you have to wait four weeks to get the drug out of your system before you can introduce a new one. It's a very painstaking process.

Here I was trying to fight off this terrible black, all-encompassing depression, and every time I tried a new medication that didn't work, it was yet another disheartening blow – another hope dashed.

When you are an adult, taking part in a process over a year or two doesn't feel like a big slab out of your life, but when you are doing this from the ages of 15 to 17, it is a huge proportion of your life to spend suffering and to feel like your life is wasting away. You see all your friends going out, attending parties, having relationships and enjoying themselves. Life was passing me by.

All this happens while you are at home being miserable, and people are blaming you for being the author of your own predicament.

The side effects of the medications for me were horrific: one of them completely neutralised all of my emotions and turned me into an automaton. I still knew who my family were, but I felt neither love nor hate, I felt nothing for them. I was a robot, and that was worse than having unwanted emotions. I'm such an empathetic person, and here was a monster who was the complete opposite of who I truly am.

There was another drug that made me suicidal. By that, I mean I wanted to act on the suicidal thoughts that were always there, but under control. I just exploded and everything became much worse than it had been. Yet another drug 'helped' me gain 20 kilos in a month. It was like I was eating fat. That particular medication was not one I took regularly, but it had been a sort of emergency-only medication to calm me down when I became really intense. It did calm me down. Another medication had other side effects, including trembling hands.

Although medication kept me alive during my very worst moments, nothing worked for any length of time. If anything, I felt the drugs made things worse over those 15 months. I didn't blame anyone for this. It had been explained to me that there was no one answer and we would just have to give a number of options a go. At the time, I did have hope that we would hit on something that was right for me and would take away the pain. And it was something to do; a project I could throw myself into.

However, with each failure, my hope diminished. For a lot of the time my situation really did feel hopeless. The only thing that kept me alive, apart from whatever natural resilience I possessed, was my innate desire not to hurt anyone, and I knew my death would cause immeasurable suffering to my family. Their constant care and determination to get me better through all my terrible moods showed me how much they would lose if I were to end my life. I must admit there were many times I genuinely believed that my long-term life would continue to cause more pain to my loved ones than my short-term death. Luckily at these indescribably hopeless moments medication prevented me from acting on those beliefs.

I had never doubted my family's love. Whatever was behind my depression, it wasn't a sense of being unloved. Knowing what my death would do to my mother, nanna, brother, father and the rest of my family, I couldn't do that to them. That was the only thing that stopped me. Better to punch walls and contain the physical harm to myself.

Ironically, I treated my family very badly. I would scream, yell, rant and rave at them. I abused and swore at them. Couldn't I see that this was hurting them too? In my own naivety, I took my family for granted. This was the safe, secure place where I could let off steam and vent my worst behaviour.

My mum copped the worst of it. I would tell her that I hated her. I probably blamed her for my problems and it was always aggressive and abusive screaming. Horrible stuff. It was all these feelings I had about myself and needed to get out of me. I would go into my room, slam the door, stuff something under it so my mother couldn't get in and hurl a petty cash tin against the door so it would make a frightful noise, rip the cupboard doors off their hinges and upend my bed. My poor mum had no idea what was going on inside my room but must have imagined that a demon had been unleashed.

On and off, this pattern of bad behaviour had been happening since late primary school. In the face of this, how did my family – and my mother, in particular – respond? They kept reinforcing how much they loved me and that I would get through it. Always. Thank goodness they took that tack. Had there been reprimands, punishments or tough love, had my mother done anything other than what she had done, if she didn't trust her gut feeling – I wouldn't be here now.

I had grown up in an environment where friends and family were all together in a cohesive social network. There were no divorces and no rifts. I took this lucky situation to be fact, not realising that family and friends could choose to be otherwise, that they could leave you if they wanted to. Family is not fact. Family is not guaranteed. They could have abandoned me, and goodness knows, I must have given them pause for thought on that after some of my tirades. Just the continual, unrelenting misery of being with me must have been so wearing on everyone around me.

At the time, I had no idea how fortunate I was. My belief that your family will be there no matter what, did not accord with the experiences of many people I met during my treatment. Some of those fellow sufferers of depression had been left to struggle on their own. And for some, their families had been the cause of their illness. If I found dealing with depression an almost insurmountable ordeal with my great army of supporters, how would these lonely people ever survive?

Whenever I was at the top of the stairs or on the cliffs, there would be a millisecond when the thought of jumping flitted through my mind. But it was just that. I never wanted to hurt anyone.

My darkest moments were at night, always at night when everything was off and I was alone and I'd cry myself to sleep. I'm not a religious person by any means, but on several occasions when I was feeling very low, usually when another medication didn't work, I would lie in bed and cry and I would pray to something that I didn't believe in. And I'd call it the 'God of all the Universe' ... I didn't know – I just spoke. I definitely believe there's something there that forces you to have hope. I wasn't even praying to get better, but just to know what it felt to be happy again.

These prayers would always end with me saying, 'Even if I can't get happy again, just make sure my family and my friends are happy without me. If you can't help me, make sure that everyone else around me is happy.' So I was contemplating the possibility that I would not be around. If the depression could not be resolved, my existence did seem untenable. I knew that the praying was illogical, but I needed to plead my case to someone or something

mum, i wish i was dead

that had greater power than me to sort things out. Of course, I was seeing my psychiatrist during this time but I knew there was only so much he could do.

My mum was a great emotional support in this period. We always had an open, good relationship. The basis for this goes back to one conversation I had with her when I was younger, perhaps a 14-year-old, when she laid her cards on the table. After starting at the new high school, she sat me down and said: 'Adam, I know your friends go out drinking and I know what they do. I know that they lie to their parents, saying they're sleeping at this person's place, the other saying they're sleeping at that person's, and they go off wandering the streets. God forbid something happens to you and I get a call. Please let me know where you are. I won't bother you, but at least I'll know where you are if you need me. And if you do need me, don't ever hesitate to call under any circumstances.'

When she said that, she was acknowledging that I would likely get up to mischief as any young boy might, but that was not her biggest concern. She'd rather that I was safe. She made me realise that being open with her was the most important thing, and I didn't need to fear her reprimands or intervention in my life. As well as establishing a basis of trust between us, she managed to remove my need to rebel. If she already knew that I might do some naughty things and wasn't trying to stop me, then part of the motivation to do those things was removed.

She said: 'I don't agree with it. I'll never support it. I'll never give you money for it and I'll never buy or supply alcohol. I know what you guys do; I'd rather know of it, than put my head in the sand. Now you know how I feel about it.'

Ever since that moment, I felt that no matter what the situation was, I could always tell her. I wasn't in any trouble, and it took away the burden that if I told her something I'd be punished and made to feel guilty. She said, 'I know you, and trust you to make the right decisions'.

I think that one conversation allowed me, several years later when I was going through all this, to be as open as I was. I made a promise to her that if there was anything wrong, I would always tell her. 'Please let me know and I can get help,' she said.

We also developed a language to speak with each other. Whenever I was pouring my heart out and she was there listening to me telling her how bad everything was, she'd keep saying, 'It's okay, it's okay'. Once, sitting on my bed, crying my eyes out and hating everything, she was trying to reassure and comfort me. She had her hand on my back, saying, 'Adam, it's okay; it'll be okay'.

I yelled, 'It's not okay. This isn't okay!' I associated being okay with being good, with everything being alright. I said, 'No, it's not okay. Stop saying it's okay!'

With tears in her eyes, she said, 'What do you want me to say?'

And I said, 'All I want you to do is hear me'.

As soon as she changed her words to 'I'm hearing you, Adam, I hear you', that took away the anger of hearing that word 'okay', because I knew it wasn't okay. Changing her response from 'It's okay' to 'I hear you' made the world of difference. I just wanted someone to hear me. That's all I wanted.

Seeing the psychiatrist was not as much help to me as my relationship with my mother. However, I think the psychiatrist helped her, because he was able to explain to her what I was going through and how to cope. Over the years, we had both learned how to deal with it: I would tell her exactly how I felt and she would give me space. Initially, that was fine, but no matter how much she tried to rein in her emotions and not to burden me with her feelings. I could still see the pain in her eyes whenever I said 'I can't keep living like this, I need it to end'.

During that period, dad was not a big emotional support. My relationship with dad was always a bit strained. He didn't find emotional communication easy, and would rather 'do' than 'say'. Because my rationale was clouded by the depression, I couldn't interpret the 'doing' normally. I needed words; I needed the emotional support. Although with hindsight, sometimes saying nothing is better than saying the wrong thing.

When I'd sound off about dad to mum, she'd make excuses for him. She'd always say how much he loved me but that they just have different ways of showing it. She'd point to the lovely home and lifestyle we enjoyed, but that's not an argument that makes sense to a kid. You don't know anything about employment and earning an income. You don't appreciate how long it takes to earn $50, let alone how much it costs to run a household. You just know that it's there.

mum, i wish i was dead

At the time, I didn't understand his distance at all, but with hindsight I realise that his version of caring for me was to work hard. And he did that, absolutely. I knew that whatever help was out there I could access it. However, increasingly I was wondering whether there was anything out there that could save me. You can't wave a fistful of dollars in the air and be guaranteed to get what you want. Money isn't a shield for mental illness. Depression can and does affect anyone, whether rich or poor. It is indiscriminate.

However, I can say that my dad's financial buffer *did* smooth the way for my next emergency.

As part of the trial-and-error medication process I'd been on, that drug which had caused me to become suicidal sent me over the deep end. I'd become extremely agitated, to the point where I went to my mother and said, 'I'm not feeling safe. You need to get me to a hospital.'

It was a Sunday night and the situation was dire. My mum knew that after my experience in the public hospital with my leg pain, I wasn't keen to go back there, but this was an emergency.

We arrived at the hospital at around nine at night and I was admitted. They knocked me out with a sedative and I was pretty well out of it for the next day. The hospital didn't want to discharge me on the Monday because I was still dopey, so I stayed on for a second night.

On Tuesday, my parents had managed to get me into a private facility on Sydney's north shore. That was certainly something my father's hard work had enabled me to do. I didn't understand it at the time, but having private health insurance made this difficult process that little bit easier. Most people get their insurance for possible physical injuries and illness. But the importance of it covering mental illness is equally as crucial.

The first time at this private clinic was for a three-week period as an inpatient. The idea was to have me under supervision for that time, away from home, from school and all other stresses. This way I could focus on my one problem and take part in group therapies. We could also find a medication that worked in a controlled environment where my responses would be under watchful, health professionals.

On the day I was admitted I went into the ICU (Intensive Care Unit) rather than the general wards. This is standard practice for a new admission so they can be accurately assessed. The ICU is monitored by the nurses' station and you can't walk freely in or out – you have to be buzzed in. The rooms are isolated behind glass so that the nurses can keep a watch on you. There are blinds you can close for privacy, but not for any prolonged length of time.

At the admission into the ICU, anything that could be construed as a cord with which you might try to take your life is removed from your possession. That included shoelaces, belts, my shaver lead and my mobile phone charger. I had to give the phone to one of the nurses to charge because I couldn't do it in my room. For the same reason, scissors, files and any other sharp objects were also taken away. In ICU, I was on suicide watch, and I remained there for a couple of days before moving into the main wards.

That was my first experience of such intense restriction and observation. It was very odd and confronting. However, I did feel safe because I knew nothing could happen to me. In a weird way, I was not worried about the future.

Being in this situation created what I like to call an optimism effect: you're going to hospital, the health machinery is working, I'm going to feel good, I'm going to feel good … In your head, you think you are going to feel good. It's as if going through the motions promises the right result.

Once, during a turbulent time, I remember an appointment with my psychiatrist when I told him that everything was good. It wasn't, but I thought that if I told him everything was good, and if I told everyone else around me that everything was good, and I told myself everything was good, I could maybe trick myself into thinking everything *was* good. But that didn't work. It lasted only for a very short time. Everything I tried, whether medication, types of therapy, self-delusion … if I felt good, it wouldn't last any longer than a week or two. Nothing had longer lasting effects.

***

I was the youngest in the general mental illness area in the clinic. There was another area just for eating disorders and the majority of those being treated there were female and some of them were around my age. The only time you'd see them was at meal times in the communal cafeteria.

Everyone smoked. I would have smoked cartons of cigarettes passively just by being in their company. Everyone would sit outside, talk and smoke, and I didn't want to stay inside by myself. I never touched a cigarette and

mum, i wish i was dead

never would, even being around it all, due to the promise I made my nanna when her sister died from lung cancer. I always like to keep my promises.

A lot of the time we actually spoke about the different medications. We'd sit around and ask each other, 'What do you have?' They'd say, 'They think it's bipolar, but now they think it's a bit of schizophrenia', or 'I suffer from anxiety'. Then someone would ask, 'What medications are you on?' 'Oh, I used to be on that but it had terrible side effects. Now I'm on this one and it really works.'

And that was good because it allowed you to be aware and to go to the doctor and say, 'I was speaking to someone about it. Why don't we try this?' The doctor would say, 'Just because it worked for someone else, it might not work for you, but let's explore it further.'

Or if someone said, 'I was on that and it made me gain a lot of weight', I'd think, you know what, I don't want to go on that medication even if the doctor suggested it. So it was very interesting. The openness and honesty, without judgement, was extremely refreshing compared to what I was used to.

There was a lot of group activity that went on and we all shared our stories of how we got there. Group therapy was an integral part of the clinic. Everyone was reasonably open about what they'd been through. I was certainly open. As soon as we'd get into the room I was ready to talk. I was finally among people who actually understood my stories. I thought, 'This is fantastic!'

The feedback I'd get from them was very confusing. They'd say, 'it's really brave of you to speak up about this. I wish I'd had the confidence at your age to do it.' Or they'd say that they wished they'd had the awareness of what was happening to them at my age. The catchcry was always, 'With hindsight, I realise that I was going through all this when I was younger'. They had managed to mask it with alcohol, sex, drugs, relationships, work or in some other way, and finally they'd ended up where they were.

These were all different people from different walks of life: teachers, lawyers, doctors, husbands, wives. They were very accepting of me, even though I was much younger than them. They mothered or parented me because of my age.

Surprisingly, being a teenager in what was essentially a ward for adults with mental illness was not a hardship. I felt the most comfortable I had in years. No one was saying naive things like, 'Try to look on the positive side.'

Or throwing it back in my face and saying, 'How can you feel this when you have everything?' They could genuinely empathise with my position. They'd listen and then share their stories. It made me so much more aware that other people were suffering like me. It was the first time I didn't feel alone. I actually felt quite 'normal'.

It also made me realise how lucky I was to have my family. Some of the patients were there *because* of what their family had done to them.

I felt very safe, very accepted, and in a way I felt at home there, more so than I had in a very long time.

There were, however, two minor incidents that occurred during my stay. The first was a misunderstanding with one of the nurses, which stood to jeopardise my continued stay at the hospital. The nurse, an older woman, believed that I was threatening her and reported me. Luckily, a male nurse intervened and organised a mediation session with her. I was totally unaware that I had caused any offence and certainly had no intention to do so.

When we were sitting in the meeting room, the woman was very flustered and I was thinking, 'What the hell is going on!' We were both rattled and distressed by the situation. I was trying to justify what I had said and to explain that it was taken out of context, that it was never meant that way. I was apologising profusely. Luckily it was resolved or I would have had to leave.

The other incident caused me no grief at all, but it did upset my mother. She rang to speak to me one night and I wasn't in my room and the staff couldn't find me. They had no idea where I was.

'What do you mean you can't find him?' my mother implored, panic rising in her voice. 'My son is only a teenager, he's depressed and he's in your safekeeping. You can't just let him walk out onto the street.'

At the time, I was sitting on the front steps outside the clinic, having a quiet moment to myself, and totally unaware about the anxious search for me taking place inside.

Though my frame of mind had improved enough for doctors to let me leave the clinic after three weeks, my emotional state returned to my usual one, once I was back home.

***

mum, i wish i was dead

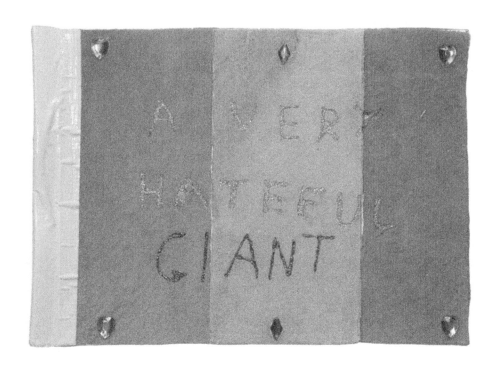

A VERY
HATEFUL
GIANT

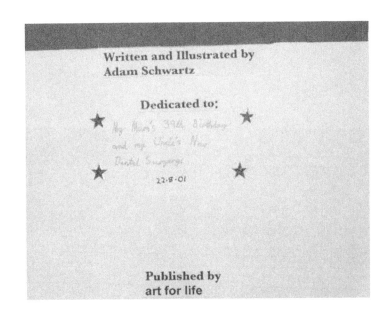

Written and Illustrated by
Adam Schwartz

Dedicated to:

My Mum's 39th Birthday
and my Uncle's New
Dental Surgery.

22·8·01

Published by
art for life

Once upon a time
there lived an
EVIL
monster and the
monster's name was
Hateful.

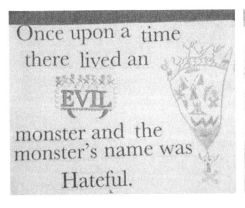

He lived on top of
a very lovely town
and the town's
name was ...

Lovely Ville and everyone in Lovely Ville was lovely and happy having a GREAT time and enjoying their life.

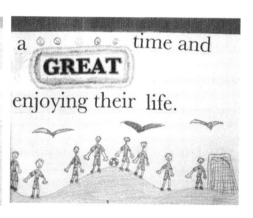

But one day Hateful got very angry because everyone in Lovely Ville was having a nice day (not that Lovely Ville ever has a bad day) So Hateful was angry right, so then Hateful's house had steam coming out of it so Lovely Ville's people knew that Hateful was very angry and then all the people in Lovely Ville went up and tried to make Hateful **lovely** and one person said

"That's impossible" and then Hateful picked up the person and swallowed him in one gulp.

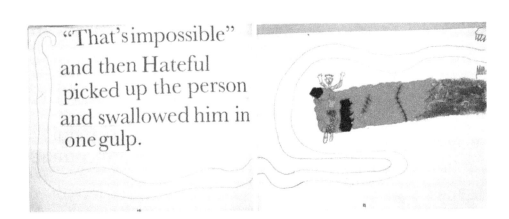

And everyone

gasped !!!

And everyone tried
everything to

make Hatefull
lovely and

then suddenly

Hatefull stopped and
then he went

bezzerk.

He started shaking and
jumping up and down

and then he stopped

and coughed up the man he had swallowed in one gulp and said, "I'm sorry everyone, but thanks"

Hateful said to the man he swallowed "because you turned my angry switch on to happy."

And so Hateful changed his name to Happyful and played with everyone in Lovely Ville. And sent them all a letter which

said:

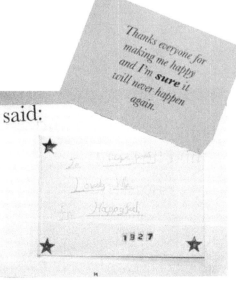

Thanks everyone for making me happy and I'm **sure** it will never happen again.

To: Lovely Ville

From: Happyful

1927

And when all the people in Lovely Ville received the letter they all yelled out

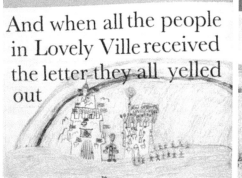

"Thanks Happyful !"

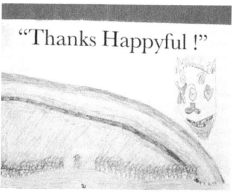

The

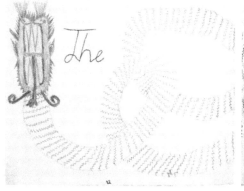

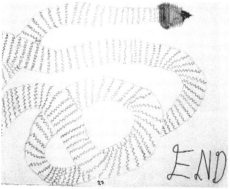

END

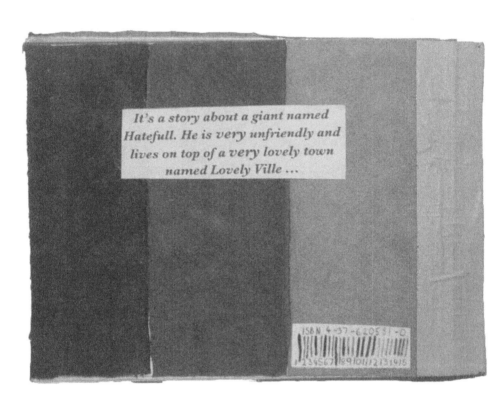

It's a story about a giant named Hatefull. He is very unfriendly and lives on top of a very lovely town named Lovely Ville …

ISBN 4-37-610531-0

Date: Wednesday, 15 August 2007 (aged 16)

From: Anne
To: Hugh

Hi Hugh

Adam had a bad night last night. Everything seemed OK
and he knew about the blood test this morning. When
I went to give him his medication at about 9.30pm,
I knocked on his door and he yelled at me to go away
and was very aggressive. He said he isn't taking
his medication and is sick of it all. I could hear
that he was tapping away furiously on his keyboard.
I tried again at about 10.15pm, although not as
aggressive, he told me to go away and he wasn't taking
the medication. I said I would leave it at his door.
He was still up at about 1.30am tapping away at his
keyboard ... So Adam hasn't had the *medication* and I
am guessing he didn't take the *medication* either.

What do I do re medication and any suggestions in
general ...

As I think he will be asleep most of the morning, I
will go to work for a few hours.

Thanks
Anne

Date: Tuesday, 11 September 2007

From: Anne
To: Hugh

Hi Hugh

I had a long chat with Adam last night (at his request) as he is extremely sad. He wants to be like and do what every other 16 year old kid is doing. He says he has no self esteem or confidence and doesn't want another summer where he is embarrassed to go to the beach. He wanted it all to be fixed by the end of the week.

After chatting, Adam has said I should contact the personal trainer he had before and discuss diet and exercise looking for quick results. The trainer is coming today at 10:45am. Adam will also take the *vitamins* on a regular basis. He has been offered a job with a lot of flexibility which I am hoping he will consider and he will continue helping his art teacher. I will work towards getting some routine in Adam's days ... little steps.

Adam is quite adamant about not taking medication and not having ECT.

I was wondering how you felt about Adam not seeing you at the moment as he isn't taking medication and he would concentrate on his physical fitness etc. I thought I could send you weekly/fortnightly updates on his progress. Also, we are happy to pay for any time you take in your consultations with us even though you may not be speaking with Adam direct.

For a bit of info re last two weeks. My mum had a right pneumonectomy (?) (right lung removed) last Tuesday and is coming home today. Adam went to Adelaide last Monday and came home on Friday (earlier than anticipated). Adam spent yesterday at St Vincents emergency (had to get an ambulance to take him) as he had symptoms that could either have been due to a high temperature, encephalitis or meningitis. Thankfully all is well and it is likely it was a nasty virus.

Please let me know how you think we should progress.

Regards
Anne Schwartz

Date: Sunday, 23 September 2007

From: Anne
To: Adam

Hi my beautiful boy

I know things are hard for you at the moment and I am trying not to hassle you.

Would you please let me know if you would like me to invite a family for dinner this Friday night ... maybe the *xxxx* family or someone else you may like. The sooner I know, the easier it will be to arrange

something. I also understand if you would like to
keep it quiet and simple.

Also I know you are trying to do things your way,
but I don't know if this includes continuing with the
personal training sessions with *xxxx*. He assumes he
will be coming on Monday. Please let me know if this
is OK or if you want me to cancel it.

I love you
mum
xxx
PS - it is OK to respond by email rather than talking
to me

Date: Thursday 27 September 2007

From: Adam
To: Anne

im done fuckin listenin to u and every1 elses lies

nothing ever gets done wat i want to help me ...

thigns only get done that impromised will work and
make things better if I jsut hang on n go through hell
for months on it 2 see if sumtin happens but guess
fuckin wat nothing u or any1 else has told me to do
wich ive done has helped the slightes

im done listenin to your shit and your empty promises

im doing things my way n im done givion a flyin fuk
wat u or any1 else thinks cause theres nothign about
me to be proud of i dont have a liufe worth living

there is nothing good in my life

i dont have a reason to wake up

i could go on about stuff u have already heard and
ignored

im pathetic and dont have one single thing in my
favour

so im gonnna start smokin as of tomorrow cause well
ppl lose wieght and

might stop me form wantin to die so bad

and if that doesnt wokr well i will jsut go and kill
myself

jump off my balcony so u can cum home to a dead body
might be nice

but im done tryin things that might help or have a
chance to the one thing i

wanted i cant fukin have and u have no idea how i feel
so dont u even dare

thinkin u have a slight clue

and dont bother tryin to speak me out of doin anythign
because ive listend

to yours and every1 elses bullshiut from ya mouths ove
rn over n its never

helped

u wanna get my attention do something actiopsn speak
louder then words

so since nothing works for me n the one fukin thing i
asked for jsut one!!

one of my suggestions i cant get o no wait i can but i
have to wait over

amonth b4 i can even get an appointment jsut to be
told they cant do anythign for another 6 months

so basically if this doesnt work ill die 16 years old
and u can guaren dam tee that i promise u i will die
unless my life get substancially better cause im not
waitin for u or any1 else to help me cause no1 has
ever made things better

no1 has ever made me happier so im done waiting for
sum1s help so ill either die of cancer wewn im 40 or
die wen im 16 from depression so

yeh hard chocie to make but theres just no other
options

so u enjoy knowing that

mum, i wish i was dead

Date: Friday, 28 September 2007

From: Anne
To: Adam

Adam, what is happening at the moment is beyond what dad and I have the knowledge or experience to help you with. This hospital is one of the options ... the other option is to get the community based 'crisis team' which is attached to Prince of Wales Hospital involved. They will come here and speak with you and assess the situation.

I love you.
mum
xx

11

A Shocking Last Resort

The 'crisis team' would be a Plan B if I couldn't bring myself to go to the North Shore clinic. But as it turned out, I was happy to be admitted. While I was in the North Shore clinic, it was an eye-opening experience to be with so many people who had my disease. We could compare notes and see the different paths that had brought us here. I was keen to find out what things they had tried, with and without success, as there might be something for me that I didn't yet know about.

One of the treatments I learned about was electro-convulsive therapy, or ECT. Mention ECT to most people and they will reel back in horror. If depression is stigmatised, then ECT is one of the most controversial treatments for the depressed. Visions of the 1975 movie *One Flew Over the Cuckoo's Nest* come to mind. But that was a different time and there was some understanding that patients were being subjected to this treatment against their will.

For me, nothing could be further from the truth.

When I had returned home after that first private hospital visit and mentioned ECT to my parents, they set up an appointment with the doctors to find out more about it. I was doing fine after my discharge but we thought it best to explore ECT in case that was a path I might one day pursue. We spoke to the head honcho of ECT in Australia about the different versions of the therapy and what would most likely be used in my case. And then we left.

The dose for ECTs varies. There are several different bandwidths. There are unilateral shocks to one side of the brain, bi-lateral to both sides and bi-frontal. The shocks also vary in length of time they are administered, so they can be brief or longer.

As you step up the dose, you are prone to more side effects and longer memory loss. The more prolonged the treatment, the worse the memory loss. But over time, once you stop having ECT, your memory does improve.

Some of the people in hospital had progressed to the stage of bi-frontal ECT, and they had forgotten their families. The memory loss can be very, very bad.

It wasn't until some months later, when my condition had deteriorated again, that the option of ECT came up once more. Apart from my parents who supported my decision to proceed, no one wanted me to have ECT, but I was adamant. There was no doctor who had said to me it was a good idea. Everyone was telling me about the side effects, including the risk of extreme memory loss, or saying that it may not provide any help and it also meant that I'd have to be in hospital for at least two months.

When I opted for ECT, I was 16 years old and desperate. Nothing else had worked. I felt this was my last resort. I had reached the point where if the ECT didn't work, I would end it. There had been nothing else that would stop me – I was ready to go. Although I can now see I was suffering from depression from a much younger age, at the time all I knew was that I had fought for two years and that was long enough in my books.

If there was a chance that ECT could save me, I thought, bring it on.

In the nearly two years since I'd been given the diagnosis of depression, there hadn't been a long enough period of feeling good in which to re-energise. I hadn't been able to regroup and keep fighting. There hadn't been a month that I could say I'd been happy. I was completely depleted. I'd made the decision that this was my last resort. The threat of memory loss paled against all this. Since my life lay in the balance, no side effect was going to deter me.

ECT introduces controlled seizures as electric currents are passed through electrodes placed on your head. It's used to treat severe depression, bipolar and schizophrenia, but exactly how it works is a mystery. It's a treatment that has been shown to be safe and effective over more than half a century, with only short-term side effects and no permanent effect on the brain. Only recently has there been a slight swing back in the popularity of ECT. It is given so rarely to children and teenagers that there is not much by way of statistics or information for me to read about.

As the date for my therapy came closer, I started to get cold feet. My biggest fear was the memory loss. If I forgot my family *and* the ECT didn't work, then I'd be left with nothing. My parents encouraged me to stick with my original plan and tried to quell my anxiety. I was scared, and that may have been exacerbated by the fact that I'd gone off medication.

Date: Thursday, 4 October 2007

From: Anne
To: Hugh

Hi Hugh

For an update … Adam seemed to pick up a bit after last week's drama. He has been seeing some friends and going out a little bit. He had another "episode" last night … sick of it all, wants to move so no-one can contact him, nothing works, just wants to be happy etc etc. We will see what pans out. I continue to encourage admittance to the private clinic and ECT and he won't trial meds again at this point in time. Only wants ECT if bilateral … I think there is a lot of fear involved in going for ECT because of memory loss so in his irrational state he doesn't really see it as an option … might try and get him to speak with the head of the department again.

　　　　　　　　　　　　mum, i wish i was dead

Does the clinic know Adam may be going there?

Thanks for all your help with the Crisis Team. They were very helpful and I now know what the procedure would be. Hopefully, we won't have to call them.

Enjoy your holiday.

Regards
Anne

When the decision had been made to go ahead with the ECT, I'd already taken myself off my meds. Straightaway, I went cold turkey. I felt that the drugs had slowly stopped working for me after my hospital visit and I was done with doing what I was told to. This probably wasn't the best idea as I knew from past experiences that stopping so suddenly could have serious side effects; nonetheless I was fed up.

I was hospitalised at the private clinic so that I could receive the therapy as an inpatient, although there were others receiving the treatment who would only turn up for their sessions and then return home.

My regime, as it was explained to me before the treatment began, would be three sessions a week on Mondays, Wednesdays and Fridays, every week for up to two months with assessments along the way. I very quickly became used to the drill. Firstly, you had to remove all metal jewellery. No rings or watches allowed. Then you would exchange your regular clothes for a hospital gown, be weighed and have your blood pressure taken, before taking a seat in the waiting room with the other patients.

I would talk to those in the room with me, hearing their stories and being invited into their private lives. One very attractive woman, probably in her early 20s, was an unfamiliar face. I remember striking up a conversation by saying, 'I haven't seen you around here before'. It turned out that she was receiving treatment as an outpatient because she couldn't afford to live in at the hospital. This was one of those times I realised how lucky I was with my family and my father's determination and hard work to provide me with the healthcare I needed. This young woman said all her family members, several brothers and her parents, were getting extra jobs to afford for her to have private healthcare. I hadn't needed to give the cost of my healthcare a second thought.

Before the ECT, you would be anaesthetised. The needle would go in and the doctors would ask you how you were: 'Yeah, good, okay'. Then they'd ask you to start counting backwards from 10. '10 … 9 … 8 …' and between 8 and 7 I'd always take a really deep breath. It was probably the thing I looked forward to most – getting the anaesthetic. It was an amazing warm feeling rushing through your body. Then I'd wake up several hours later, with a dry mouth and a bit of gluey stuff in my hair where they had put the electrodes to monitor my brain. Otherwise, I was fine. That was it.

The ECT was, almost from the start, surprisingly successful and I was doing so well that they took me off it sooner than the doctors had expected to. I was waking up and feeling much, much better. But as soon as the treatment ceased, I started going backwards, so I returned to it and finished off the course.

It wasn't just me who could sense the improvement. Everyone could see that my mood and behaviour had improved. In the latter stages of my stay, I'd started using the gym at the hospital. I hadn't even thought of doing any exercise before that. I also changed my diet. It was like my brain had kicked into gear. I knew what I had to do because I had been exercising and was quite fit for the 12 months prior to when the depression started. So I did it. I started walking on the treadmill, which developed to doing some weights, then jogging on the treadmill and eating better. My fitness cycle was getting healthier while I was undergoing the ECT.

My health, my personality and everything else improved as a direct and immediate effect of ECT. And I was happy. That was it. I'd started to feel good. I could see how I was, and I looked forward to getting the ECT because I thought: 'This works. It works!'

During this time I was told that I might need ECT once a month for the rest of my life. I remember thinking, 'I'd much rather get a zap in the head once a month than have to take medication every day. What happens if I miss the medication, or I want to go drinking with friends and the medication and alcohol don't mix, or I have to endure the side effects of medication for life?' Getting zapped in the head once a month seemed a better option than living with the repercussions of medication every single day.

As I finished the course of treatment, the hospital staff said that I should book in for the next course. I told them I was happy to wait until it was required. They agreed, on the proviso that I continue to see my psychiatrist and psychologist, which I did.

I was 16 when I had ECT and I have not needed any medication or ECT since then. However, if I ever dipped again and needed medical intervention – and there has been only one occasion when I was really bad and came close to it (and that one episode was either brought on by jet lag or Seasonal Affective Disorder) – ECT would be my first port of call.

I'm not saying I'd recommend it to everyone. It is very invasive and I've seen the detrimental side effects it can have. However, I was one of the lucky ones and it was my salvation.

There is definitely a place for ECT in the treatment of depression, but it is used as a last resort. It was my last resort.

With the treatment successfully over, I was ready to go home. But it wasn't only me who had changed over the past couple of months; home had changed too. I would be going back and trying to fit into a family with a big hole. One of my parents had left.

12

An Absence at Home

When I was hospitalised to receive the treatment, I knew I was going to be there for a prolonged length of time. That didn't bother me when, after a few sessions, I realised that the ECT was starting to work.

One day, my parents came to visit me in hospital together and they asked if we could go into a private room because they wanted to speak with me.

I assumed it was going to be good news because it felt just like in the movies when parents sit their children down for a talk to tell them that they are about to get a baby brother or sister. I actually thought they would tell me that mum was pregnant again, even though I knew that wasn't possible. So maybe they were going to tell me that they had won Lotto or they had made some major purchase. It couldn't have been further from the truth.

When I think back on it, I imagine that I was there with a big smile on my face. It was as if I were ready to share in their good news and was preparing to say, 'I knew that's what you were going to tell me. Fantastic! That's really great.'

Ironically, even though I was depressed, they didn't seem upset. They sat me down, and they were holding each other's hands. They started off by saying that they still loved me and that this doesn't change our love for you.

My mum was doing the talking, and I felt as if she was still building up to some big positive news, such as a new baby, until she said, 'Dad and I are separating'.

Everything just paused for a while. It didn't seem real and I couldn't believe it was actually happening. My thoughts were always buzzing around in my brain but all of a sudden everything in my head stopped. I was completely in shock. My parents always seemed to have had an easy and comfortable relationship with each other, so this came totally out of the blue for me.

The first thoughts I became aware of were about Nathan, who was 13 at the time. I felt very protective of him. Regardless of what I was going through, I didn't want him to feel like he was alone. I knew that my parents' separation would devastate him, and that's all I was concerned about. Even though I wasn't conscious of the fact that my own problems must have had an impact on him, I was fully aware that this would crush him. I got up and left because I only wanted to see Nathan and speak with him.

Unbeknown to me, Nathan had really wanted to see me too, especially after he'd learned about the separation, a week or so before I was told. He couldn't understand why my parents were able to visit, but not him. He figured that even if I was in a bad way, he is my brother. Surely he could only make things better for me, not worse?

He was also concerned about how I would cope with news of the separation, but had resigned himself to the fact that he wasn't allowed to see me because of the strict scrutiny I was under.

He was surprised when he received a text message from Mum saying that I was coming out of hospital, just for a brief escape, to see him. Mum asked where he was and said she would bring me to him at 4pm. He was down by the local beach so we met up at the headland nearby, just the two of us. It was very incognito.

In spite of all the rules and regulations surrounding my treatment, which required that I not leave the hospital, I'd managed the break-out because I was determined to see Nathan. I would have said something like, 'Let me see my brother ... or else!' They knew how serious I was and that this wasn't an idle threat.

Nathan describes our meeting that afternoon as being surreal. While usual life was going on around us, Nathan knew that I'd been in high security hospital care, receiving ECT. Very shortly I'd be returning to that closed unknown world away from him, the hospital wristband I was wearing was a reminder of that. He says I was very flat, perhaps a result of a course of ECT that morning.

We spoke for more than half an hour, and managed to reassure each other. Yes, our parents were splitting up, but we were going to get through it together.

I was also very angry with my parents, as the following email from my mother to my psychiatrist shows …

Date: Wednesday, 24 October 2007 (Adam aged 16)

From: Anne
To: Hugh

Hi Hugh

Nathan has had two meetings with *xxxx* the psychologist. The first was the day after we told him that Tony and I were separating. Nathan seems to be doing OK so not sure when he would like to see *xxxx* again.

Adam has had six sessions of ECT. He seems fine - just with headaches afterwards which they give him painkillers for. He was very angry when we told him about the separation (the day after his first ECT). Initially didn't want to see either of us. Now it is just Tony he doesn't want to see. He has changed his mind a bit about the whole situation. Initially thought that we didn't try hard enough, then angry at the timing, now angry at Tony not just about the timing but has said to Tony that he was only pretending when it appeared they got on. He says that he is not unhappy about the separation. I think he isn't sure about what he feels and isn't dealing with it too well. He has been very supported while at the clinic. Hopefully it will all settle down before he comes home.

Not sure what the balance is re hospital as I haven't spoken with the doctors again. They seem to be primarily liaising with Adam. Tony has been in touch with psychiatrist at the hospital to see if she has any suggestions as to how he should deal with Adam but nothing is forthcoming.

Tony and I are getting on well, which I think has helped with Nathan.

Hope you had a good holiday.

Regards,

Anne

I probably wasn't really able to take it all in or to show much concern for my parents. I don't even think I asked them why it was happening. Part of it was a protective mechanism. I knew that I was starting to get better and I had to hold on to that. I couldn't let the process that had given me this one ray of hope be derailed.

Also, I was still a child, used to focusing on myself. People often refer to teenagers as believing the world revolves around them. In my case, this natural tendency to self-centredness was probably intensified because so much of my energies, and those around me, were consumed by the depression. There wasn't a lot left for anyone else.

While I was cocooning myself from feeling the effects of my parents' split, it was nevertheless a complete surprise to me. There hadn't been any 'writing on the wall' that I had been able to read. Again, the depression and solving it had been all-consuming, so you might think that the signs were there but I hadn't seen them. I didn't see the sadness or emptiness in my mother. I never saw her crying and I was unaware of her pain. Nor was I aware of any frustrations from dad. My guess is that my parents had gone to great lengths not to show any of their problems to me.

Nathan, however, had seen it coming, though I only learned this recently. He says that our parents told him one morning to be at home by four in the afternoon because they both needed to speak with him. 'I knew exactly what they were going to talk about,' he says. 'For months, those two had said, "Oh, we are going tonight to see a movie", but they were going out somewhere else.' From the first time they said it he knew they were going to marriage counselling.

Nathan says, 'At home, they were both under a lot of pressure. Mum had a lot of emotional stuff on her plate with Adam and her own mother's ill health, and dad had a lot of work stuff on his plate. It was very, very busy. I thought the break-up was inevitable; it was just a question of when. Nevertheless, I was still heartbroken when it happened.'

Nathan's concern was how he was going to fit visits to both mum and dad into his own busy schedule. 'I wanted to see as much of both of them and didn't want to favour one over the other. I realised seeing them separately was going to take up a lot of my time and I didn't know how I was going to manage all of it. I was a bit confused about that,' he says.

Incredible to think that he was only a kid and had felt this huge responsibility for his parents and to treating them fairly!

Though he had been at home to witness our parents' relationship finally deteriorate while I had been in hospital, Nathan showed far greater perception than I was capable of at the time. My depression had affected my ability for rational observation, so if there were signs, I don't think I would have been able to pick up on the stuff that had been happening between my parents.

Later on, when I asked them why they had told me in the middle of the ECT therapy, they said it was because I was in a safe place. I was in hospital, and I couldn't have done any harm to myself once I was established there.

In hospital, the separation didn't feel real. I was living in a completely unnatural environment and my life was somehow on hold. There were none of the daily interactions with family members around the home, such as breakfast in the kitchen, meal times at the dining table, watching TV or family outings. So it wasn't until I packed up my bags and left hospital that I felt the awful truth of our changed situation: Dad wasn't at home anymore. He had his own place.

Although I didn't know it at the time, my parents had been going to marriage counselling – as Nathan had guessed – before the split. They were determined to sort out their relationship with each other. Well, at least try to.

Mum says that she had harboured a resentment of my father for years, feeling that he had left her to raise us children on her own. He was never around to fully take part in the parenting. Their ways of expressing love were different: hers was to be involved in our lives and his was to work hard and provide us with a comfortable lifestyle.

She says that she also felt judged in her mothering role. My dad would ask her if I'd managed to get to school of a day, and she would read that as if my non-attendance was a failure on her part. Of course, he actually just wanted to know how I was getting along, but my mother had interpreted it differently.

The advantage of the counselling was that my mother got to hear how my father was feeling too. She thought he didn't realise that she felt like a single mother most of the time. Now she learned that dad was feeling like the unnecessary fifth wheel. He felt like he didn't have a place in our house. He could see how well mum was coping and that she had lots of support from her parents and family friends. Also, when he was at home, he and I would often be in conflict. Ultimately, I think he left because he really did love us as a family and felt he was causing us a great deal more stress by being at home.

The timing of his departure was really bad for mum with me just starting the ECT. She told him that if he left, he wouldn't be coming back. It would be over.

I was a lot closer with mum at that stage. She was very much the emotional support and had been there for me all through the terrible years that had finally brought me to the hospital for ECT so I automatically took her side. For a very long time, maybe months, I didn't want to speak to dad.

We'd been planning a family holiday to Bali before I'd gone into hospital. It would be in the long Christmas break. Now, what would we do without dad? It was decided by my parents that the trip should still go ahead, but without dad. Until the holiday rolled around, dad had kept contact with us by dropping around now and again and having some meals with us. It was clear that even though he was living elsewhere, he still wanted to be part of the family. However, what kind of family holiday is it when the father doesn't join in? That's when it hit home that things had definitely changed.

While we were overseas, mum was ringing my grandmother every day. Because the New Year was approaching and my grandmother wanted to ring my dad to wish him a happy year, she asked my mum if she would mind her doing that. 'Of course you should ring', my mum said.

When they caught up with each other by phone the next day, my grandmother said she'd asked my father if he ever thought about getting back together with my mum. It had been about two months since he'd left our home. His response was, 'There's not a day I don't think about it'.

My mum had softened and realised that he had softened too, and when we returned to Sydney she started talking with him about the possibility of him moving back home. He was very nervous about it because it had been a very huge thing for him to leave and he was worried that if he came back it may not work out. My mum said, 'What have you got to lose? You won't know unless you try.'

My father decided he'd better have a talk to Nathan and me about the possibility of being reunited. He came and asked us what we thought and whether we would like him to come back. We both said that we hadn't been consulted about the separation in the first place so why bother to seek our opinion now? What difference would our thoughts make? We told dad that it was up to him.

In April, six months after he had walked out, thankfully he walked right back in. My mother's threat that she wouldn't have him back was just that – a threat. She claims she said it because she was so angry at the time and she hoped it would stop him from leaving.

In spite of my worries about Nathan's reaction to the split, he was very strong about it – at least publicly. My situation had no doubt affected him and our parents' separation would have been the straw that broke the camel's back. He was holding back on his feelings. I don't think he was comfortable sharing it with me because he didn't want to make me feel any worse. He kept a lot of that to himself. He didn't want to blame me or add any further stress to my situation. For my part, I just wanted to make sure that he was okay. Maybe he sensed my need that he be protected, and so he reassured me by appearing not too upset.

It was a very sad time, and especially so for him because he was as close to dad as I was to mum. Nathan didn't want any of his friends to know about the separation. I think he was embarrassed about it.

I had been worried about Nathan but not my parents because they were both adults. And I needed my mother's support to get through. I didn't realise it at the time, but I was selfish. I didn't try to get all this attention, but I needed it. I think you have to be a bit selfish in order to survive. I had to focus on myself, especially when the therapy was working. I had to concentrate on the good that was happening. I wasn't strong enough to take on board other problems and I couldn't allow something else to bring me down.

I was going to do whatever it took to get back to my old self. My parents' separation didn't feel like it had an effect on me either way. However, in retrospect, I think my depression had affected them.

At the time, I think I did ask if the separation was because of me, and they both reassured me that it wasn't. But a part of me didn't believe that. Years later that question resurfaces and I now truly believe that I was a key factor that caused their separation. I know I put a huge amount of pressure on their relationship. It was a really weird feeling for me. I didn't know what had happened. They said that they had grown apart and it was a mutual decision and they just both reassured me how much they loved me.

My parents will admit now that, while my depression was not the cause of their separation, it put an extra pressure on their relationship. Any person who is ill – and depression is an illness – puts extra pressures on the family, loved ones, relationships and any other support networks.

With all the days that were sad and full of anger, this was a different thing. For the first time there was a reason to feel sad. And that was weird for me because I was so used to having these emotions with no logical foundation.

But a lot of good came from the separation. It made our family much stronger. I think we all benefited in some way.

While dad was living apart from us, my mum definitely encouraged me to see him and I started to do that. My dad loved me very much but I just hadn't got along as well with him as I did with mum. We began getting closer when we started going to the gym together. We both had to learn a lot, especially how to communicate with each other. I had never spoken with him about my emotions because he wasn't an emotional person. He saw himself as the financial provider.

I'm sure that my parents decided between them that dad would work and mum would stay home or work part time and look after us; however, at the time I wasn't mature enough to realise this. Nonetheless, I wanted and needed that emotional person in my life, not just the financial one.

The separation had an amazing effect on everything. It lasted for six months and it forced dad to appreciate what he had and to learn how to open up. The separation was probably due to a lack of communication. Dad supported us by removing any financial worries so that mum could do whatever she felt was best regarding my treatment and not be constrained by the costs involved.

But mum wanted someone to help her make those big decisions about my care. She felt like she was bearing the sole responsibility. My dad understands that we love him and we want him to be part of our lives. We have all had to grow, make changes and learn how to better communicate with each other.

My parents are back together and stronger than they've ever been. I have a relationship with my dad now that I never thought I would have when I was younger. My parents have a better understanding of each other than they had before they split up. There is no doubt in my mind that it has brought our family as a whole closer and our individual relationships with each other are better. It had a very positive result.

mum, i wish i was dead

13

Home for Christmas

While in broad terms, ECT had turned my life around, there were still occasional lapses in the next couple of months when I would become sad or angry. How much of this was still about unresolved issues from the past six years and how much a response to my parents' separation, I have no idea. But it would be wrong to paint the picture of my return home as an altogether rosy one.

Yes, I was much, much better, but emails from the time covering the Christmas holidays and my 17th birthday show there was some way to go ...

Date: Tuesday, 18 December 2007 (four days before my 17th birthday)

From: Anne
To: Adam

```
Hi Adam
I can see that you are in a bad mood ... please let me
know if I have done anything to upset you or if I can
help in any way.
```

The show tonight starts at 9:30pm. If we leave at about 8pm we can have a coffee beforehand or if you prefer we can leave at 8:30pm. Just let me know.

xx

Date: Tuesday, 18 December 2007

From: Adam
To: Anne

im in a bad fucking mood cause im so fukin sick of everything

i dont have shit all no more... ive lost fukin everythign i had

i feel like fukin shit cause of everything.... i dont have a life anymore

i dont have any real friends i dont have anything

i dont hvae sumtin to wake up for... yerh i keep tryin n tyrin to no avail

i have 0 self confiedecne i have 0 self esteem i dont have the ability to do anything

all i want to do is leave and get as far away from this place as humanly possible

im done with this "family" i have n im deff done with the "friends" that i have

mum, i wish i was dead

i sick of it and everytime i get one thing sorted 10 more fucked up messes pop up

i was ready to come outta hospital but i wasnt ready to come back here

i cant be around here anymore cause i odnt ave anythign left here except bad memories

hell i dont even have any1 to have ova 4 my bday... i dont even have anythign to celebrate

and u have no idea how i feell... infact no1 does

caus eim 16 n i have no life.. i have no1 that likes me n i have no1 that cares

n im done wasting my energy on it

im not going wiht u tonight n im not gong with u to bali

right now i dont want to do anything right now all i want to do is leave here and get better n ready to see ppl my own way

not aroun other ppl not around any1 just me doin my own thing so i can get better

so i can get ready to come back to this place and these ppl

i feel like shit... and ive felt like shit for awhile

and thanx to that fuckin moron [name removed] i
thougght i was gettin a treadmill so i could get
better

but no i was waiting n felt good n was hopful n
optimistic but him being a stupid fukwit gives me
false hope

i coulda been wakin up early every morning doin
excersise and feeling gr8 again but no .. i dont
feeel fukin compfortable enough to do it at the gym
or outside or anything

i really dont cause i have 0% of everything left

so i dunno wtf im gonna do anymore.. ive lost my hope
my optimism my everything

so i dont know.. i dont have a fucking clue

all i know is im done n i want tot get wat i want

im not going away with u n nathan im not going out
tonight....

there will be a treadmill in this house... and i dont
giev a fuk how much it costs

take money out of my bank for all i care

thats gonna get me better and thats gonna give me
confiedence back

so thats wats going to happen one way or another

mum, i wish i was dead

Date: Wednesday, 30 January 2008 (aged 17)

From: Adam
To: Anne

i cant look at your and speak about everything because
i see how badly it hurts and upsets you

i havent felt this way in a long time, and i havent
had this much rage inside me for longer

i cant be around people when im feeling like this

dont say once your around ppl your will feel
better, because i have such rage inside me that i
could smash not just my fists into a wall but through
it, along with my head

i hate feeling like this, i hate that i cant use my
brain, i dont want to be around people asking me
questions, i dont want to be around people in the
state and feelings that i currently have

i look in the mirror and i see nothing, not one bit of
anything i can be proud of anymore

i dont feel hopeless surprisingly, i just need
something about me worth waking up for

i refuse to go back to my depresion, only reason i got
out of bed

cause everythign was going great before this school
thing was going to start

i was excersising losing weight, but like always with
me theres a hell of alot more to lose

i have had such bad experiences and loss of everything
i no longer have any confiedence to do anything that i
enjoy, i havent been to the beach in years because im
so self consiece

i feel bad enough as it is and returning to a place
were i once thrived, to find that not only cannot i not
even use my mind but the simple fact is the friends i
thought i once had i really never had to begin with

i just want to wake up infront of the mirror and feel
good, see something, anything! Good and let me make
this very clear, im not proud of myself because for
once i thought a plan i had would actually work, but
as usual with me and everythign i aim towards it falls
through adding to making things operfectly clear i
have not one single clue about anything anymore

and finnally the only reason i got out of bed is simply
because i cant go back to were i was with my life im
not going to rot in my bed im going to have a life
worth having and thats horrible because even with all
the good in my life, i still feel exactally how i do
and just for the record i want to go to school i really
do, just hate whats become of me and thats basically it

from your failure of a son

adam

mum, i wish i was dead

Date: Wednesday, 30 January 2008

From: Anne
To: Adam

To my beautiful boy

When I look at you I see a person of amazing strength who I admire and respect. You have had a lot to deal with for a person of your age which I cannot truly understand. I do see your sadness, frustration and anger. I see how you try to protect us from what you are feeling. I see how you still strive to achieve your goals despite the setbacks.

I ask questions so that I can try and understand and help you.

I am here to support you. I need guidance from you on how best to do this.

I am here for you whether you prefer to send an email or speak directly to me.

I love you.

Mum

xx

14

An End to School Daze

ECT, my wonder treatment, had removed the fog of depression but replaced it with the fog of forgetfulness.

My memory loss was minor by comparison to those who had forgotten who their children or siblings were, but it did interfere with my return to a 'normal' life. Post-hospital, the plan had been for me to go back to school full-time, and repeat Year 11. This would mean finishing just a year behind the kids who had started school with me. There was also discussion about doing Pathways at my school, a program that allowed you to complete Years 11 and 12 coursework at your own individual pace. This meant that I could do half the curriculum load one year and half the next, to ease me back into my studies. However, I really didn't want to be 20 years old and just finishing high school.

So I went back to school and all seemed fine. My original buddies were in their final year and didn't quite know how to react. They kept a friendly distance and it was kind of weird. But there was a much more disconcerting problem: I couldn't for the life of me remember the work I had to do. I had severe short-term memory loss.

I would remember going to school, but I had no idea what I had done during the day. No idea what I had for lunch, no idea about any of the details of my day. I'd remember the general outline, but nothing specific.

After one of the first days back at school, I came home in the afternoon and showed my mother my exercise book, saying, 'Mum, I was obviously in class learning all of this, and I've written it down, but I don't remember doing it, and I don't remember any of it.' It was very scary.

It was also frustrating because I knew intellectually that I could do the work but I would sit at my desk, unable to do it. Maths was the worst because you needed to learn new stuff every day. One day you'd learn the basics then each class would build knowledge on the previous lesson, and I wasn't taking anything in.

Needless to say, the final years of high school are all about remembering. At no other point in your life is there as great an emphasis on memorising everything you do. If I couldn't recall whether I'd played handball at recess, what hope did I have of committing to memory the lines of Shakespeare or the rules of a quadratic equation? School was not going to work for me. I lasted there only a fortnight.

Leaving the classroom again proved to be one of the hardest decisions I had to make. It felt as if I was giving up on my future. Once I had thought I could take up any profession I wanted. Whatever I chose to be, I could achieve by putting my head down and making the grades. I'd always been a high achieving student, so doing well in the HSC like I'd done in other exams and gaining entry into my preferred university course, wouldn't have been a problem. But now it was. Maybe I wouldn't ever get to university. Maybe I'd be a high school dropout.

We didn't know how long the memory loss would last. As it turned out, it was only three months. I had already left school by then, because it had been a complete waste of time being there. Actually, it was worse than that, because attending as an almost mindless student was undermining my self-confidence. I knew I was smart, had found school easy and actually enjoyed it in the past, but this was not the time …

My memory improved slowly, day by day. It wasn't as if one day I couldn't remember anything and the next day I was fine. After the three months, my memory had returned completely. It was 100 per cent as it had been, as good or as bad as the next person.

One of the slightly amusing things about my memory loss – only in retrospect – was that it made me extremely gullible. Since I had forgotten to be cautious about taking on face value what people said to me, and because I often couldn't trust memories of my own experience, I'd believe whatever

I was told. No matter how implausible the story being told to me would be to others, I'd think, okay, that's cool. I believed everything.

On a plane trip to our family holiday in Bali, my brother and I were playing a game of cards. My mother and brother said something unbelievable, but my response was just to smile in complete bewilderment and say, 'Oh, okay'. After all, if they were telling me this, it must be true, right? Both my mother and brother asked, 'Did you not know that we were being sarcastic?'

I had no idea at all. I said, 'Are you being serious?' I was completely unaware of how naive I'd been. It was sickening for my mother, who was quite anxious that I could be taken in by unscrupulous people.

My plan to use my brain, as I'd always done, and get into the university course that I wanted – all that had been taken away from me. For the first time in my life, I had no idea what to do. In the end, I wanted to get healthy.

Leaving school at 17 allowed me to focus all my attention on getting healthy. I went back to the gym and continued to see my psychologist. The ECT had provided a great springboard to recovery but I still had a long way to go.

I started with a new psychologist once I had completed the ECT. I was reluctant at first as the psychologist was a man. I much preferred the idea of relating to females. Mum had to book the appointment and drag me along. She had gone to visit him beforehand, to give him some of my background and to vet him to see if he would be right for me. It was very important that mum did that, to make sure that he was okay for me, because if he wasn't – if I had a bad experience first-off – it would have hindered the chance of my seeking out another psychologist.

I'd recommend that approach to anyone who is the carer or a family member of someone seeking help: do as much of the groundwork as you can. You probably know the person better than anyone else and can ease the whole process.

So, for what seemed like the umpteenth time, I told this psychologist my story. Over the years, I would say, 'I can't be bothered telling my story to someone else again'. That was the hard part, retelling your story, everything that has happened, the same bloody thing, over and over again, to a new doctor, or psychiatrist or psychologist. It was painstaking.

I started seeing him once a week and the initial treatment was cognitive behavioural therapy (CBT). The CBT was all about retraining my thought

mum, i wish i was dead

processes, helping me to let go of all the thoughts that were causing me to be plagued by anxiety. When I was walking in public I was still very paranoid and would feel that people were ridiculing me. If someone three tables over from me in a restaurant started laughing, I thought they were laughing at me. I was still seeing the world through the same eyes.

I'm not keen on CBT because it wasn't the most effective therapy for me. You basically have to think yourself out of how you are feeling. CBT is about trying to rationalise the situation to reduce the anxiety. I liken it to having a splinter in your finger; it doesn't bother you all the time but whenever you use your finger, the pain is there. CBT can lessen the pain, but it is still a band-aid solution because it doesn't address the real cause of the pain; it doesn't remove the splinter.

We tried other therapies as well, including Eye Movement Desensitisation and Reprocessing (EMDR). This therapy tries to get you to uncover the cause and then deal with it. It gets to the splinter and rips it out. That means, whenever you are faced with the triggers that used to bring on the pain, there's nothing remaining to hurt. That's what it did for me, and it has helped me greatly. It's still a therapy I use today.

EMDR gets you into a dream state using a couple of methods, such as listening to a beat move from one side of a set of headphones to another, or following someone's finger moving from left to right, or holding a vibrating object in each hand and the vibration moves from one hand to the other. The result, basically, is that your eyes start shifting from side to side, as they would when you are dreaming.

The idea is that, when you are dreaming, your subconscious is resolving all the emotional issues of the day. By inducing this state during counselling, you can be guided to address long-term emotional problems that the conscious mind has not recognised.

Apparently, the theory behind EMDR is that a person who is suffering from an unresolved trauma may, in the face of further distressing experiences, find their usual coping mechanisms overwhelmed. The aim of EMDR is to process memories of the trauma, thereby reducing its lasting effects. It pulls the metaphorical splinter out.

This was the therapy that in the not-too-distant future would provide a moment of clarity for me – an epiphany.

15

Addicted to Exercise

While it had been a hard decision to leave school and give up on my dreams of a career, for me, at the time, it was about being happy. Happiness trumps everything else. The rest could be dealt with down the track …

As well as regular visits with my psychologist, the other area of my life that had to be addressed was my body. I'd been struggling with my weight for so many years and the smorgasbord of medications I'd been sampling for the past two years had exacerbated my problems. At my worst, I was obese, weighing in at 120 kilos.

In truth, my weight was an indication of my emotional state. When I was bad, I was fat. It was a pretty straightforward equation. Even as a little kid, I was chubby when I was depressed, and a relatively average weight when I wasn't. Now that I was well out of my terrible rock-bottom dip, I was nowhere near that super heavy record weight I'd achieved before the ECT, but still my appearance was bugging me.

However, I have to confess that my real motivation to lose weight was not about getting better or being healthy. I figured that my emotional wellbeing was under control and heading in the right direction. The catalyst for going to the gym was because I believed that if I looked better, someone would like me. Romantically. Possibly even love me.

My friends who were girls would sit there and say: 'I wish we could find a guy like you. You're so nice … blah, blah, blah.' Well, if I was so nice, why was I being ruled out as boyfriend-material? I didn't want to like someone and end up being 'just friends'. Logically, I thought if my personality is so fantastic, it must be a physical problem. So my idea was to go to the gym and train to look good, thereby removing any impediment to my love life.

The exercise had started already in the hospital when I was receiving ECT. Back at home, and with no school studies to interfere with my time, I had plenty of hours to devote to my new project of getting trim and building the body beautiful.

I wasn't a stranger to exercise. During those really dark years of my depression, one of the nicest things to happen was a weekly outing with family friends to a football stadium on Saturday mornings where we'd train together. The dad would come and pick me up, every week. He was completely committed to our outings and it was the one thing I could rely on doing, no matter what else was happening in my life. After training, we would meet up with his wife and kids, who were a year above and below me, for breakfast. It was one of the most consistent and enjoyable events of that time and allowed me to build up a great deal of confidence.

It had been a low-key gym, not a show-off gym, and I liked that. You don't get the people who are 'roided up'. You don't get people who are massive dudes and don't eat any food, just protein shakes and food supplements. At those gyms there are women who have had plastic surgery and they are all shiny and pretty. They are very intimidating for someone who is self-conscious and doesn't know what they are doing. When I go to these places and I see older people, very young kids or people who are overweight, I admire them for not being put off.

Eventually, the mum introduced me to a larger gym, part of an international chain. I still kept up Saturday mornings with the dad at the non-threatening stadium, but gradually managed to feel comfortable in what had been the more daunting gym with all these brutes walking around and all these polished people.

The consistent routine of gym and breakfast with their family made such a significant difference to my life. At the time when I felt like people were around me for sympathy, they made me feel so included and supported that I knew they actually wanted me around, especially when they didn't have to have me. Even as my health improved, those Saturday mornings were the starting point that led to my career in physical health. It made me realise how lucky I was that my family had such good friends who cared that much about me, as well as how important exercise was to my emotional health.

Now, after the ECT and having left school, I was at the gym every day and doing exercise classes every morning. I said to myself: 'This is my life, this is my work, this is my school – I am getting better'.

My deficient memory wasn't a problem at the gym. During a fitness class you were repeatedly told what to do, and I wasn't going to lose my way home.

I couldn't drive, so my dad would drop me off at the gym at 7.30am. I'd delayed learning to drive because I had enough on my plate and didn't want to add the pressure of driving lessons. I wanted to wait until I was at a stage that I felt comfortable doing it. There had also been the memory issue. I didn't feel it was safe, so there was no way I was going to take the risk.

At the gym, I'd start with a spin class, which is basically a vigorous workout on an exercise bike. Since the bikes are in a fixed position, the spinning refers to the whirring of the pedals. You normally begin with a warm-up, then adjust the pedals for greater difficulty, sometimes peddling in a seated then standing position, as if mounting a steep hill. After 'spinning', I'd move on to use the other equipment for a couple of hours, and return home by bus of an afternoon and help mum around the house. I'd still see a psychologist and everything else, but that's what my life was.

Over the course of five months, I ended up losing more than 35 kilograms. I couldn't believe it. The first 20 kilograms came off easily. When I eventually plateaued I got disheartened, and my psychologist actually suggested I look into the low GI diet as a possibility, and once I made my mind up to try it, it was the easiest thing to do. Instead of eating icecream and putting on a couple of kilos, I'd resist, knowing how beneficial it was to steer clear of those foods.

And so the last 15 kilos came off, and I stopped weighing myself. I've never touched a set of scales since, because I realised I was anchoring my happiness to a number. Going to the gym and exercising made me feel good and gave a purpose to my day. I loved it and I was doing it for me. That was another big change because I was doing something that was good for myself. I wasn't doing it for another person anymore. The initial motivation of romance went. I was doing it for me.

mum, i wish i was dead

Everything was good and, three months after the ECT, my memory had come back.

With exercise, you have to start off slow, eventually getting used to it and building your strength and confidence. And I did. I really got into it. There's no doubt in my mind that I got addicted to exercise; it sort of creeps up on you. I would notice that I'd feel frustrated if I didn't exercise and exercise chewed up all my time. When I was unable to exercise, for whatever reason, I'd be aware of all the negatives about not doing it. However, I never thought about the many positives of exercise when my routine wasn't being interrupted.

I was over-exercising like there's no tomorrow. It was ridiculous. I'd reach the point where I'd do my first spin class at 7.30am and then I'd go straight on to another spin class at 8.15am. Now spin classes are hard, and I was going all out with them. It's a bit over the top to do two in a row.

Or I'd get on a treadmill and run for 20 minutes at a speed of 10 km an hour. I've got little legs so that was pretty fast for me! Then I'd do my 8.15am spin class for 45 minutes, then I'd do another 20 or 30 minutes on the treadmill, then I'd go and do an hour of weights. Way too much, but that's what I made my life.

I'd reached this extreme after I'd lost the weight. I wasn't keeping up this manic pace to keep losing weight any more. I did it because that's what I did during the day since I wasn't at school and I wasn't working.

In spite of getting healthier and healthier, both in mind and body, I still had a lot of issues about the way I looked. It's very strange because even though my body had changed drastically, I was still seeing the world through the same eyes. When I looked in the mirror, I couldn't see the huge transformation. I was obsessing about being overweight in the same way as I had when I was depressed. I still didn't like the way I looked.

I'd walk through the shopping centre and people were looking at me, and all these thoughts would swirl in my head that I was unattractive and that people were laughing at me.

My dislike of my body had been so bad that I even considered plastic surgery or liposuction after I came home from hospital. I begged my parents to let me go under the surgeon's knife too. I'd always been conscious of my large chest and felt I had man boobs. Under my constant hounding, my mother organised a consultation with a surgeon.

We spoke at length, and I'm so glad I didn't get anything done. But that's how bad I was: a teenager wanting to undertake surgery – not for medical reasons but to improve appearances, believing it would make me happy. At the time I thought that this was the only option I had to feel better about myself. And I was contemplating this radical treatment *after* I had lost weight.

I still couldn't look in the mirror, couldn't go to the beach, couldn't talk to or approach any girl I liked. If someone had complimented me, I honestly thought they were saying it from pity and I took offence.

There was always this belief that if I looked good, everything would be better. I absolutely believed it.

Date: Sunday, 1 February 2009 (aged 18)

From: Adam
To: Anne

hey, just me

yeh i'm pretty sure you have noticed i've been pretty out of it lately

just letting you know im feeling pretty shit

i dont know why exactally but ive been starving for no reason, i feel self concious, i have no motivation for anything anymore, i feel really sad and lonely atm

ive tried to still do things and see people and keep busy but it doesnt seem to be helping

im not sure where im at or wat i even have to talk about, but yeh

mum, i wish i was dead

i just wanted to let you know were im at with
everything

i know your always helping and trying but i dont know
wat can be done to help atm

im thinking if its like usual it will just take time,
but its been a few days now so im not sure

i feel overwhelmed, but im not sure wat is making me
feel that way.. i dont know wat i want and i dont want
to go backwards

i hate feeling like this so much, because its a
horirble thing to fele and it drains me... im
startiong to over think things again too

dont ask me wat i want to do becaus ei honestly have
no idea

i really am tryin mum   ... i hate wen i try n
things go backwards... i really feel so awfull atm

i try to pick up n motivate myself wne sum1 calls,
but even this arvo wen *xxxx* rang im like losing the
energy to even care

i dont want you to worry, but i did promise u i would
always let you know where im at

. hopefully ill pick up soon.. but if not.. well yeh

thanx, love you

xx

16

Personal Training

Now I had to turn my attentions to the next phase of my life. What was I going to do with myself as far as a career was concerned? I'd depended on my parents as all children must, but my needs had been more demanding. While all my friends were making the move seamlessly from high school into university, and into professions that many had mapped out years before, I had taken a side step out of that safe, preordained existence. I'd had to. But it was time to join my peers back in the world.

From what I'd learned on my own journey, was there something I could share with others?

Over the past year, constant exercise and fitness had become my daily fare. In fact, I had become a gym junkie. There wasn't very much I didn't know about the inside of any exercise facility and I was a convert to the benefits of keeping fit and healthy. I had swapped classes at school for gym classes, and here too I'd been an excellent student.

But without completing high school and so not obtaining a Higher School Certificate (HSC), I needed to learn what options were available to me to train for a job.

I went to see a careers adviser and she was fantastic. I was asked all the right kind of questions and she knew about all the education requirements and certification needed to enter every field.

The adviser suggested the health industry, mentioning at first the possibility of becoming a nutritionist. Then personal training came up as an option, and that's the one I decided on.

It seemed reasonable that my total absorption in exercise should eventually lead me to become a personal trainer. I believed if I could lose the weight myself and overcome my challenges, then I could help so many other people. I was used to using my head, and now my memory had returned, I wanted to get an education in how to teach those skills to others.

With a definite plan in mind, you'd think it would be easy for me to focus on the goal. However, I was feeling emotionally wobbly, which could have been brought on from a recent overseas trip (jetlag or Seasonal Affective Disorder), and was questioning this career path even as I started out.

Date: Tuesday, 17 March 2009

From: Anne
To: Nick (my psychologist)

Please see email below that Adam sent me. Since the email, he has restarted working towards completion of his personal trainer certificate, has one client and exercised more frequently.

I have also requested a new referral from Hugh.

Adam will see you tomorrow at 5pm.

Regards,
Anne

Date: Wednesday, 11 March 2009

From: Adam
To: Anne

i dont know what to say exactly but i just feel so lost

i know what right, i know wats good for me, but at the same time i honestly dont know why but i dont care and me not caring is makin me feel worse.. even though i know i should care i just feel like ive failed and i dont even know wat i feel like ive failed

maybe i fele like ive failed at life.. but im only **18** so i dunno anymore.. a big part of me wishes we never went away cause everythign was planne dn sorted n going down the path i wanted

n now being back i cant get back onto that path... no matter how easy every**1** is making it for me

i feel so much pressure to do the things i know that r right.. but honestly i dont think it worked last time

i feel like i worked sooo dam har dn it hasnt really got me anywhere... im struggling not to compare myself

i feel like i dont deserve things.. n that i dont really have anything in my life... wich is stupid cause i know i do

mum, i wish i was dead

```
but my logical head isnt connecting with the
physical feelings.. all my "issues" r from how i
feel.. not my logical self and besdies that my heads
been all over the place... im juts finding eveyrthign
so frustrating.. and no theres nothing u can do
because if i knew what to do it would have bene done..
and talking about this i dont know wat to talk about..

im not feeling depressed.. im feelin lost and
confused, and thats makin me feel useless and
frustrated\\]

i dunno to be completely honest but yeh.. thats me
atm.. just letting u know so u dont worry

have a good day at wrok

love u xx
```

Over the next few months, through a certified fitness institute, I completed the intensive Certificate III in Fitness and then the Certificate IV in Personal Training, allowing me to work as a trainer.

I initially started training others at the gym, five days a week, but that proved to be too heavy a load for me. I still needed time for myself. So I moved to working three days a week – Monday, Wednesday and Friday. That allowed me to get used to my new reality as I was still working through a lot of issues, learning how to be around people, socialise and hold conversations.

On my days at the gym, I had about a dozen personal clients who came to see me. When I wasn't training one-on-one with them, I'd be managing the floor and conducting boxing classes and all other sorts of classes for the gym members. This was a very small, boutique gym, so it was full on.

I had always been the person to whom people came for advice, so my new position as a trainer was a sort of extension of that. I enjoyed helping others and people seemed to feel comfortable discussing their issues with me, in spite of my relative youth.

Apart from my natural inclination to talk through problems with others and be supportive, my experiences with counsellors during my depression gave me further impetus to adopt that role.

I did everything with a passion. When I first went to the gym, another trainer was leaving so some of his clients were handed over to me. They were older people and, as you would expect, a little reluctant to work out with me as I was only 18 at the time. I even looked younger than my years. Although they were hesitant at the start, it wasn't long after their first few training sessions with me that they began to increase the frequency of their gym visits. If they had been coming twice a week, they quickly converted to three times a week. Those initial clients never left me. I didn't lose a single client in the whole time I was training.

I got on with most people and those I didn't get on with, I learned how to deal with. I learned a lot of skills generally, and met a lot of people. My training style was very different to the majority of other trainers. Just as I didn't believe in weighing myself, I didn't weigh any of my clients. I had realised that anchoring my happiness to a number on a scale was not only irrelevant, but also harmful. If you are losing weight every week and doing all the right things and all of a sudden you plateau or gain weight, you feel disheartened and bad about yourself.

At certain times of the month, women put on between one and three kilograms just in body fluid. Fluid retention can also depend on how much salt you've been consuming. The scales can also be reflecting last night's indulgent dinner. And different scales can give you different reading. It's defeatist to regard one measurement at one point in time as a mark of your worth. If you are still doing all the right things, such as eating well and exercising, then you'll feel great. You need to concentrate on the big picture.

Most of my clients would come in saying that they wanted to lose weight and tone up. The majority were definitely interested in looking good rather than being healthy. I was always open with my clients about what I'd been through. I would say, 'Look, that's fine if you want to lose weight. But I don't want to weigh you. You can go home and do what you like, but I don't believe that's important. I'm training you to be well.'

I was always interested to know why people had decided to come to me and I would always manage to get to the reason behind their visits. Why did they want to exercise?

For the older clients it was really just giving them something to occupy their day and maintain their health. They wanted to be social, to get out, to do something. For the younger ones, usually they'd just been through a breakup. They wanted to get fit and attractive so they could go back out there and find someone to be with again. Surprisingly, that was the major driver for a lot of the people I saw.

If you asked the right questions, you'd always get down to it. The answer was very rarely: 'I want to be healthy'. On the surface, that might be the first response. But dig a little deeper, and that wasn't really the case.

My clients never cancelled on me. If they called to say they weren't feeling motivated, I'd say: 'Look, come and we'll go for a walk and a talk or a coffee or whatever,' and that would be the session. So much of our sessions were just talking because they had all this stuff to get through. I could understand it. I wasn't telling them what to do. I'd just listen and ask the right questions so they could get off their chests whatever was bothering them.

A great deal of it was familiar to me and everything about it was psychological. Even the super fit people had issues. The hardest part to sort out is the mind and the thought processes behind your problems. Exercising and making your body fit is the easy bit.

When clients came to me, I didn't go and pinch their fat and do the skin measurement tests you do for fitness. Because if someone is seeking you out and they are overweight, you know they're unfit and they know they're unfit. What's the point of getting them huffing and puffing and sweating just to tell them something they already know?

Every week, you can see the progress they are making. If you sense they are getting disheartened, you just say: 'When you first came in here, you couldn't do one push up, and now look how many you're doing'. I was always honest with my clients and they loved that. The feeling was mutual as I became very fond of them, too.

17

Mirror, Mirror

At the time I started training others, I was still self-conscious about my body. My psychiatrist thought I was suffering from body dysmorphic disorder (BDD). You can look in the mirror but the reflection you see isn't an accurate picture. You manage to distort it and exaggerate the image, confirming in your own mind the very worst aspects about yourself. If you think you have a large nose, the mirror shows your very ordinary one as bulbous. If you think you are fat, then no matter what weight you have lost, you still see a huge hulking body in front of you.

All my life I'd thought of myself as fat. Yes, there were times that this was the truth. I'd been a chubby kid and I'd been obese at phases during my adolescence. But now I had lost weight and muscled up. A disinterested observer would not have called me overweight. Objectively, I was healthy and my physique was good. But there is nothing objective about a person's own sense of their body image and self worth. And my view was being distorted by years of dissatisfaction with my weight.

Surely other weight losers were revelling in their new-found figures. At the gym I had seen women and men who had transformed and were now strutting their stuff, only too pleased to show off their slimmer, fitter selves. Yet I was still shrinking from public exposure, convinced that people were sniggering about me when I walked by.

I was strong and healthy of body and, having overcome the worst of my depression, I thought I was healthy of mind. Clearly, this wasn't the case. I still couldn't see myself for who I was. I saw myself for who I had been. I was living in the past.

When I had been depressed, it had been the same sense of being laughed at in public. If someone was looking at me, they were judging me and laughing. There was a great deal of paranoia that was, even at that stage, kicking in. So even though the chemicals in my brain were better and I could feel happiness and was seemingly content, those little experiences of life still stayed. Even though my body had changed physically and I was losing the weight, I was still seeing the world with the same eyes and becoming really self-conscious. Poor body image had been a constant through my childhood and adolescent years.

In my regular visits with my clinical psychologist, this was one of the major issues we worked on. Using a technique called EMDR (Eye Movement Desensitisation and Reprocessing), he was able to take me back to the first trauma that triggered this response in me of shame about my appearance.

The theory behind EMDR is that a person who is suffering from an unresolved trauma may, in the face of further distressing experience, find their usual coping mechanisms overwhelmed. The aim of EMDR is to process memories of the trauma, to reduce its lasting effects. As I described earlier, it pulls the metaphorical splinter out.

We started by talking about the latest triggers for this debilitating emotional response. For me it was the anxiety of going to the beach, talking to a girl, or having anyone look at me in public. He told me to bring up that feeling and describe what it was like.

The process then takes you back, step by step, from each situation in which these feelings have surfaced, all the way back to the initial trauma; the metaphorical splinter in your finger that has to be removed so that it can't keep hurting you every time it is touched.

Getting to that 'splinter' can take time, or it can happen very quickly. For me, it happened very, very fast, perhaps because my head is used to processing information that way now. It goes back to the event before the last one, and back, and back and back ... all the way back until the first event happened. Sometimes you get stuck and that's why the psychologist is there to ask questions such as, 'How are you feeling and are you seeing this or that?' This helps direct the thought process.

What was the starting point for me? It seems so trivial now to say, but it was something that happened when I was only seven or eight and in primary school. I was in the toilets, and a couple of kids looked over and called me fat, then ran off. At the time, it didn't upset me. Or, at least, I didn't think it did. I don't remember feeling anything. But that single moment in time imprinted itself on my subconscious and remained there.

So whenever anyone would say anything about my body, whether it was said in jest or even a compliment, I took it badly. Emotionally, I was back as my young chubby self, exposed and vulnerable in a school toilet block, the object of derision for two silly and unthinking children.

It may seem like a small thing, but that tiny splinter was embedded in my psyche. Most of the time, it didn't get knocked. But sometimes, a glance or a remark would rub against it and the hurt would flair up again. It was such a small thing that I had never noticed it. Like most splinters, you can be blissfully unaware until some passing pressure is applied. But ignore it, and the splinter is always lying in wait for you. It has to be removed to avoid future pain. Pull it out and you never have to deal with it again.

Those taunting school kids could never have imagined the effect their ridicule would have on me. But they were my splinter. With EDMR I was right back there, but while my emotions were those of a seven-year-old child, I now had the perceptions and rational thinking of my adult self to deal with the situation. I was much wiser now and understood the world much better. Who were these little rascals out for a laugh that I should give a damn about what they said? I spoke to myself and said, 'Why do I care? Why invest any value in the words of these kids?' Ever since then, I've refused to give anyone the power to make me feel bad about myself again.

When you ask those questions of yourself as someone approaching adulthood, it seems ridiculous that you ever gave a damn. However, speaking the words was a revelation and a release for me, and the effects were immediate.

I have never been so euphoric in my life. Without the splinter, I no longer thought I was fat and ugly. I wanted to take a look at myself to check out what I really looked like. As I left the psychologist's rooms and walked out onto the street, I was searching for windows and shiny surfaces to take a look at myself. It was the first time I'd actually loved who I was. And I couldn't get enough of myself.

As I write this, I know it sounds completely narcissistic. It wasn't. For so long I had hated the way I looked and this had held me back from doing the things I wanted, such as going to the beach and from forming intimate relationships. In an instant, I had realised that I wasn't so ugly to behold. Just as I knew I was a good and caring person – qualities I liked about myself – now I knew that people outside could see that goodness. I liken it to being in love with another person: When you truly love someone, they *are* beautiful to you. You *do* want to look at them all the time.

Well, I'd fallen in love with myself. I was at ease with me, after all these years. I was comfortable in my own skin. Australians are so used to being cynical that we feel we have to put ourselves down. Even when we think we are okay, we sense it is wrong to say so. We don't only cut down tall poppies, we stunt the pleasures of our own achievements, at least in public.

Instead of saying, 'I did well in those exams' or, 'I'm not bad looking' or, 'I'm a great friend', we play down our good qualities and achievements.

As I walked through the shops that afternoon, I knew when someone looked at me it wasn't to laugh, they were checking me out – in a good way! I was even checking myself out.

My family noticed the change in me instantly. It was such a novelty in those first few days that I'm sure I drove them nuts. I'd be looking at every reflective surface I could find for images of myself. At the dinner table, I would polish up a spoon to admire my face. The rebound was so extreme because the body loathing and self-consciousness had also been extreme. But it was harmless enough, and certainly boosted my confidence enormously.

I looked in the mirror and couldn't believe what I was seeing. I went and bought myself a whole wardrobe of tight-fitting clothes to show off the body I had worked so hard to achieve.

It was coming into summer and the end of the year, just before my 18th birthday, and nearly a year since the successful ECT sessions. I was ready to go to the beach again and I didn't need to cover up. A Sydney summer never felt so good.

I know how it sounds, but it wasn't coming from a place where I thought I was better than other people; I didn't think that at all. This was just about my feelings for myself. There were no comparisons to other people. That's where I always came undone, using other people as a measure for myself.

I don't believe I was doing anything wrong. I was revelling in my new-found happiness within myself. Apart from buying new clothes that were probably a size too small, I was feeling great. The grin on my face was a welcome sight to my family who much preferred the new Adam. Better a child who sneaks a look at their reflection every now and then, and walks with a spring in their step, than one who is too self-conscious to go out and have fun.

Now I realise that if you are happy with the person you are within, it should be the same with the way you are on the outside. It shouldn't matter what you look like. Being content with your whole self always comes from within. At the time, I didn't have that wisdom.

Nothing physical had actually changed. The only thing that happened was that my thoughts and view of myself had changed. Everything else went from there.

I had beat depression, lost a huge amount of weight and toned up, and now I was in a really positive head space. It had taken a great amount of effort and a lot of time to get there. I had left school and taken on the task single-mindedly, but that project of getting me better was substantially complete.

mum, i wish i was dead

18

Closer to Heaven

While I'd been getting better, my mother was at last able to stop spending all her time worrying about me and turn her attentions to herself.

She'd earned her reward, and she chose to take it by going to a spa retreat in Queensland's Gold Coast hinterland. This was no ordinary health resort, but one billed as Australia's only Eco Tourism certified health retreat. Boasting an array of awards, including winner of a recent World Luxury Spa Award for the best luxury destination spa in Australasia and Oceania, the retreat is really something special.

On her return, my mother was quite excited about the possibilities for me to get involved in the place. 'They had a work experience program … I would really enjoy it … I could further my education and explore going down the nutrition path … it would be a great place to learn,' she told me.

Her enthusiasm was met by coolness. I was basically not all that interested and with every praise she gave, my response was the typical, 'whatever'.

But I did see one advantage of her idea. At the time, I had a girlfriend and that relationship was quite disastrous. I needed to extricate myself from it and all of a sudden the idea that I might escape to Queensland seemed a good one. On the face of it, I was going to further my qualifications and progress my career path, which was a very respectable justification for my departure. But really I went up there to fall out of love with this girl and learn to be healthy.

I had always been fearful of getting into a relationship because I was afraid of heartbreak or that there would be a lack of love as a catalyst for the relationship to develop. There are many people who don't take the first steps to get to know someone because of these anxieties, but for me, a failed relationship could have disastrous consequences. I felt that an overwhelming influx of emotion could start a spiral back into depression, so I was always hesitant.

But I had met this girl and things had moved very quickly to a point where I had lost control. I was extremely attracted to her and the buzz you get from the first weeks of an intense relationship is very addictive. Almost as quickly as we had struck up our friendship, we ended it. For the first time, at least. There were all these overwhelming emotions that threatened to engulf me; there were lots of tears and sadness, which are no doubt typical for the end of an affair. However, for me there was also self-hate and suicidal thoughts. All of those destructive thoughts that had swamped me during my depression and threatened to completely destabilise me had resurfaced.

To some extent, I was prepared for this. When I had left hospital after my ECT and was getting well, part of my recovery was to establish an action plan in case I was to ever find myself in the same terrible position again. You can only create an action plan when you are well and rational. You need to be in your right mind. You have to prepare legal documents as well, giving medical and legal authority to others – in my case, my parents – to act in your best interests when you are incapable of doing so for yourself. All those documents were signed, and my parents could agree to medications, hospitalisation and financial authorisation for expenses that needed to be incurred if I was sick.

With all those things in place, if something goes bad, it would only take one phone call to the right people and doctors and hospitals will be ready to go. You'll get where you need to be, safely and quickly.

That was the thing. If I was bad, the plan was to get me into hospital, back to the private clinic where I had my ECT, and just go from there. I also had one medication, which relaxed me; in case at any time I felt overwhelmed by emotion, I could take it to calm me down. It was only for emergencies.

Basically, that's what happened when the relationship broke down with my girlfriend of the time. It all started happening on a Thursday evening. I cancelled my clients for the Friday, and managed to get through that night. I told my mum what was happening so that there would be no surprises for her, and we'd see how I was faring the next day. She also emailed my psychiatrist:

Date: Thursday, 8 July 2010 (aged 19)

From: Anne
To: Hugh

Hi Hugh

Adam has an appointment with you tomorrow afternoon.

Adam has just broken down in tears. He has been
feeling bad and sad for some time now (maybe a few
months). He also broke up with his girlfriend tonight.
Adam says he needs to do something quickly about how
he is feeling. He said he last felt like this before
he had ECT. I would agree with this after talking
with Adam it is not just because of tonight's events.
I also agree he has been struggling over the past
few months but he has been trying to manage things
using the strategies he knows. I have also given him
medication as he said he needed something to relax
and calm him. It is all I had in the house.

Would you please let me know if you are able to see
Adam earlier in the day. If you assess him with the
same conclusion as above and he needs to go to the
private hospital it would be great if we could get him
admitted tomorrow and hopefully start ECT on Monday.

Regards

Anne

When I awoke the following morning, I was still really bad. I could feel myself spiralling down into depression and that was very scary. I definitely didn't want to go back to that place. My mum made a phone call to my psychiatrist and she emailed my psychologist and the hospital. I could see that, as well as wanting to help me, she was really worried about all the good work of the past year or so coming undone. I wasn't the only one who was scared about the depression returning.

Everyone was aware of what was happening and they all were prepared to do what they could. Appointments were booked with doctors, and even though the hospital was full, they said, 'You've been here before and we'll get you in'. When you're suicidal, every minute is precious.

My psychiatrist said I should take the emergency medication. I had the weekend to get through before I could return to the hospital for possible ECT.

It had already been around 18 months since I'd had the ECT and I'd already learned from my psychologist a lot of tools and techniques on how to deal with any negative thoughts I had. I'd learned how to be rational and logical. Once the medication calmed me down, it took away the intensity of the emotions and allowed me to think straight. When you have that onslaught of emotions, you can't think clearly.

On Monday morning I received a phone call from the hospital saying, 'We can have you in; we've got a bed'. But over the space of the weekend, I had managed to turn myself around. So when the call came, I said, 'Thank you, but I don't actually need the bed any more'.

In the end, the break-up had been a positive experience for me. I had the chance to test my action plan – and it worked. But the time I spent over the weekend also showed me that I didn't need to be afraid of love anymore. I could survive it even when things went awry. Possibly the most important thing I learned from that relationship was that I was okay to love again. That was a huge thing for me because I'm a loving person and need to have those close, caring connections in my life. That momentous weekend was really the spur for going up north to reset my path.

When I landed in that tropical retreat, I was intending to spend six weeks up there on the work experience program. It is an astonishingly beautiful place, set up high on the mountain with extensive views along the coast.

Apart from the spectacular natural beauty of the setting, the resort is the last word in luxury. There are lakeside cabins, an exercise pavilion set among the trees, an infinity pool and spa sanctuary. Guests are offered everything from nature walks and seminars to yoga classes and outdoor massages against a rainforest backdrop. Much of the organic gourmet cuisine is grown in their own garden.

Arriving at this retreat was like finding heaven on earth. The whole experience of leaving home was new to me, and it was great. I loved everything about the place and I truly thrived up there.

There was so much to learn and I was devouring it, both figuratively and literally. All the information about organic food, enhanced by eating delicious samples, was knowledge that I felt should be taught to all people in the fitness and health industries. It should really be general knowledge, available to everyone.

And there was a great deal of esoteric knowledge that I gained during that time. I fell in love with being up there and I didn't want to leave.

But first: work.

The work experience that was offered was not strictly formalised. In fact, it was extremely disorganised. No one was responsible for running the program. The office staff were very friendly, and they would greet the volunteers, such as myself, on arrival, and then you'd have to navigate a course yourself, finding out whom to approach about what.

Within a week of arriving I had become very friendly with the staff. All the guests had been giving them positive feedback about me and I was generally well regarded. Towards the end of my six-week stay, one of the staff members said to me, 'What about running the work experience program?'

I approached the general manager and put the proposition to her. The advantage of having me organise the program, I told her, was that I was also a personal trainer and could step in to take over from someone if they were sick. I could run any of the physical activities and I knew the legal requirements and responsibilities. Being single, I was also prepared to live on site, so I would be available at short notice if there was anything wrong that needed attention.

She said she would think about it, and the very next day they asked me to start. They created the position and offered me the job. I had already booked a holiday so between finishing off my own work experience and starting to organise a program for others in my newly created position, I had to return to Sydney. I needed to come home as well to say my goodbyes and pack my bags for what would be a much longer stay.

I did not have the chance to say goodbye to my Sydney clients, those people who had become my friends. It had been hard to leave them the first time I made my way up north. At that time I thought it would be only a couple of months before we'd be training together again. Now I knew it would never be happening. I really did value my clients and still feel disappointed about running off without a proper farewell. I did reconnect with some of these people, much later on, and we remain friends.

My job at the retreat never had a formal job description. It was a good thing that I just knew what I was doing. I grew into the role as much as the role was shaped by me. When I first started in it, I thought I would be there forever. I was very passionate about what I did and the people who came from all over the world were amazing. It was all sunshine and I learned so much.

I was there running the volunteer program for people who were coming up to the retreat for no monetary gain, giving their time, leaving their jobs and everything else to be there and learn. I had to train two new people every week. This eventually led into running some of the fitness activities as well due to my experience in the industry.

Being busy also meant that I was not dwelling on the ex-girlfriend left behind in Sydney, and it did give me a chance to view from a healthy distance that relationship, as well as my other past relationships.

What was interesting to me is that I had always been drawn to the wrong girls. On the outside, these girls appeared to be amazing. They were usually physically attractive, intelligent, bubbly, happy people. That's also how I appear: extroverted, cheerful and self-assured. Until you get to know that I had a lot of issues, you would have no idea.

It's not having issues that are the problem. We all have our own issues and battles to face. The concern is when these issues are suppressed and go unacknowledged, only to rear their ugly heads when triggered. Always leading to disastrous results. It's hard when you can see through the mask that is worn and want to help the person you love through their pain. Especially when they're not ready to help themselves. After all, there are usually damn good reasons why issues get suppressed.

With hindsight I was attracting girls with suppressed issues that always managed to resurface. I thought to myself, 'Well I've learned this lesson. I don't need to go down that track anymore.' Then the universe stepped in and said, 'Let's test you ...'

The next week, a very pretty girl turned up for work experience. She was just my type – or was she? She was very forward and as we started talking about relationships, she began flirting with me. But more or less, I didn't find her attractive. There was no desire on my part to take this any further. The girl ended up leaving after only a week because of family issues. And I realised that the spell was finally broken.

I didn't need to take on girls with unresolved problems anymore. I didn't want complications. I didn't need to be the rescuer. No one needs that. I had been drawing girls to me who were really seeking counselling, not friendships based on equality and having fun together. I was a shoulder to lean on. I was part of the problem because I am good at being the person you can turn to when you need help. I could see through the mask and sensed the pain, so I wanted to help.

People shine at certain times in their lives and in their special area, whether it's when they are singing or painting or teaching. When people are in need of help, then I'm the one they can turn to. There's no better person to go to because nothing scares me. I can be there through the thick and thin of it all. And that's what makes me shine. I was a beacon to the needy. That's not the sort of message you want to be sending out if you are hoping to develop a healthy relationship.

At last I'd realised how unhealthy that pattern was and I'd broken that power. As a result, romance took a back seat while I was at the retreat and I was able to turn my full attention to the work at hand.

The guests who came to the retreat were there for every conceivable reason, from the desire to achieve physical fitness and emotional wellbeing to experiencing a touch of indulgent pampering.

This retreat is the shining example of health retreats and it's been around for almost a decade. You get visitors who want to lose weight, you get regulars who go up once a year or once every three months. They go to maintain themselves or just to get away and use the ever-expanding spa, which was truly immaculate. A lot of celebrities choose to go there to get away from hectic schedules and the public gaze because it is a closed retreat. You have people from all different walks of life, for all different reasons. Some people are grieving over a lost loved one and they are able to find some peace and serenity there away from their daily routine.

I could have spent the rest of my life at this retreat. While the scenery and the place were unchanging and secure, every week brought new faces and new friends. There were the volunteers under my instruction, and there was the ever-changing parade of guests, each one with their own story to tell. It was an amazing and fantastic time for me, and I feel incredibly lucky to have had that experience. I was flat-out busy, from dawn until dusk (everyone is encouraged to rise with the sun and retire early for sleep) but I enjoyed every minute.

Just as I loved to hear the tales of our visitors from around the world, when people realised that I had lost 35 kilos, they would start asking questions and my own story would unfold, over and over again. Sometimes I would find myself in a group of 20 people listening to my story as others would ask questions, then people would seek me out individually, wanting to know more. Very often, it would be parents who were concerned about their own children, hoping to get a handle on what they were going through and how they might help them overcome their problems. Occasionally, adults with their own issues would approach me, hopeful that there was a solution for them.

All these people had the same look after our conversations: 'If it was possible for this person – me – to get through it, there was hope for them'. They didn't have that glimmer of hope before. I was able to tell them that there is all this wonderful support out there if you know how to find it and where to go. I felt like they saw me as some traveller to a distant harsh land who had managed to make his way back to civilisation. It's all well and good to read the brochures and the advice to travellers, but you want to speak to someone who had made the journey and come back safely.

After having answered all their questions, the response from my 'audience' would always be: 'You've got to write a book!' Many of these people had read self-help books written by qualified experts, but they wanted something written from personal experience. What does it really feel like to be depressed and not want to go on living? When their children are suffering with depression, what can they say or do that will help them feel better? What do their words of comfort sound like to a person on the other end of the fog of depression? And, how the hell do you get out of there?

When these calls for me to write my own story came, I always managed to dismiss them. However, after a year of being at the retreat and the constant retelling of my story, I realised I had to write the book. I was ready to do it. It was time to go back home.

Even though I was away from the supports who I had relied on – my family, my friends and my psychologist – I made a new family up there. They were people I would do anything for. I no longer speak to them every day, but I know I can go back there anytime. When I do and we sit down together, it is as if I had only left yesterday.

19

Brothers

My very first childhood memory is of the day my brother was born.

It was winter and the day was quite dark and stormy. I was wearing my puffy jumper as my father took me into the toyshop. It felt like the lights were as dim inside as the light in the skies outside. Searching through the aisles, I found a green crocodile and my dad took it to the counter to pay for it. With the new toy under my arm, we headed back to the car and drove over to the hospital. And that's when I saw him, this little thing. I never let him forget that his birth is the first recollection of my life.

I love my brother, but the relationship that we have has been difficult, even at the best of times, and with my depression, we've had to struggle through the worst of times together.

We are two very different people; you couldn't find more opposite people in the world. Although we were both brought up in the same home and have the same parents, we've lived very different lives. That's not such an uncommon description of many siblings, though perhaps our divergence was more marked because of my depression and Nathan's easy-going nature.

I'm the cautious one, aware of my surroundings, always very particular with things, and black and white about what is right and wrong. I believe fundamentally in honesty. Mine was the domain of responsibility and reliability, causing no upset or bother to anyone, whether that was parents,

mum, i wish i was dead

teachers, friends or strangers. And I was loving, empathetic, caring; that's how I was, a very sensitive kid.

Maybe this is the domain of the older child. It's funny, because when I look at cousins and other family members, I can see that the eldest ones are always like me, the youngest ones like my brother.

The younger ones, like my brother, they're the ones who go and run off; they're not aware of the dangers, so they don't exist. They just do whatever the hell they want. There was no consideration of consequences or the worry they put their parents through.

At school, I was always the academic and Nathan the sportsman. Not that he was stupid, but he had to work at doing well at school, and I didn't. Similarly, doing any sport never came easy to me. It was as if we inhabited two entirely different domains: mine was the world of the mind, and his was the physical world. In our own areas, we were able to excel.

As the older brother, I felt that I was very much my own person and that Nathan just followed me around and wanted to do whatever activity I was engaged in. But, of course, that may have more to do with family hierarchy than our innate personalities.

As soon as people see us, our physical differences are obvious. Just as we are emotional polar opposites, we are distinctly set apart by our appearances. He is slim. He's fair-skinned, and when he is in the sun, he doesn't tan, he burns. He has blue eyes and pale brown hair. He can't put on muscle and he can't put on fat. He can eat whatever he wants and not gain any weight.

Whatever he is, I'm not. I'm stocky, have olive skin, dark hair and putting on muscle is just as easy as putting on fat.

When I was young, there were photos of mum at the same age and we look identical. Once, my friend came over and saw this photo of my mum and asked, 'Why were you wearing a dress?', thinking it was me. When Nathan was young and chubby he looked more like our father's side of the family. But as we grew up, we swapped over, and I now look more like my dad's side of the family and he looks more like mum's side.

As young kids, Nathan never did anything to harm me. We'd push each other's buttons and we'd fight, but it was the usual brotherly conflict. We used to love watching the wrestling on TV and we'd mimic the action by wrestling around ourselves, which caused our parents to freak out a bit. Fair enough, because I was much bigger than my brother.

So over the years I've developed a more subtle form of fighting back when Nathan incites me, rather than use my physical strength. Because that's what he wants – he wants to get a reaction out of me.

He certainly knew how to piss me off. We used to have a fish tank in the house and it was my job to look after the fish. Nathan knew to leave the fish alone because I always told him not to do anything with them. It was my stuff and he wasn't to touch my things. One day I set off to a friend's place and he took my absence as the opportunity to feed the fish.

As he'd never done it before, he had no idea about how much food to give them, so he emptied the whole container into the tank. Fish are not the brightest of animals, and rather than stop eating once they've got enough in their bellies, they'll keep going as long as the food supply remains. The unfortunate consequence is that they eat themselves to death; Nathan had killed all my fish.

I returned home the next day to discover the carnage. I was in tears over my lost fish, and furious with Nathan. Those were the things he'd do.

How did I retaliate without using force? I had to learn how to be cunning.

Before we had Wi-Fi, access to the Internet at home was via a cable. The cable entered the house downstairs, and from there the line ran upstairs, firstly into my room and from mine it continued into his room. So one way I retaliated, if Nathan did something to stir me and I didn't want to deal with it directly, instead of lashing out at him I'd simply remove his access to the Internet. I would block the cable connection exiting my room. This caused no inconvenience to my parents or to me, as we were closer to the source. Nathan was the end of the line and I'd manage to terminate the service to his station alone. He would lose his shit. That's how I managed to get back at him.

Growing up, our differences were difficult for me to accept. This probably caused a tension in our relationship. Nathan could eat whatever he wanted, but when I ate, I gained weight, so my parents would tell me, 'Nathan can have that piece of cake, but you can't have it'. Although my parents were only looking after my welfare, as a kid I didn't understand it. If there were going to be privileges for either child, didn't they belong to me as the older one? Wasn't this a subversion of the natural order that my younger, less responsible brother could be indulged in this way while I felt guilty about eating the delicious foods in the house?

It felt very wrong and unjust to me, so there was a lot of jealousy and hostility expressed towards Nathan. This was compounded by the accolades and praise he received for his sporting prowess. Australia is a nation that loves its sport, and Nathan was a sporting hero among our friends. All the families were obsessed with soccer and spoke endlessly about it; it was soccer this and soccer that. And soccer was Nathan's game. I always gave it my best, but I was never good enough. I never scaled his heights. He was good at the things that were valued by everyone else. He was the sort of person I wanted to be because it seemed like he had everything easy.

It never occurred to me that Nathan might be jealous in any way of me, but it turned out that he was, and my ease at school was something that grated on him. But you only learn these things later on. As a child, you are so wrapped up in yourself. I like to think that I am able to see from the other person's perspective, but I was so consumed with my own version of our brotherly injustice that I couldn't step back to take in his view. Kids don't, I guess. So his teasing was perhaps more than boyish bravado and possibly a chance to get his own back on a nerdy brother who sailed through his schoolwork.

When I was depressed, Nathan was amazing. He would have been 13 when I went through my really bad stuff. I would chase him out of the house and scream at him. I can't imagine what it would be like at that age to see your older brother in the state I was in, wanting to kill myself every day.

Nathan was amazing because he didn't change the way he acted or didn't do anything differently. He managed to steer his own course without impinging on me. He stayed out of the way and dealt with his own stuff, and he *was* going through his own crap at the time. Just as I had tried to spare him the burden of my misery, he was, in his own quiet way, sparing me any of the burden of being an older brother. He was getting on with things so that the energies of the house could be focused on me. And he never complained about that, or at least not to me.

He never tried to talk about the depression with me. We didn't engage on the issue of emotions: not a young boy thing. I never wanted to speak to him about it either because I wanted to protect him. I was able to turn to my mother and let her see me at my very worst. I didn't need to have Nathan shoulder any of that responsibility and I didn't want him to be exposed to it. There were times when he didn't stay at home so he could be spared my traumas. It would have been extremely difficult for him. The experience of having an older brother who was moody, unable to go to school as well as suicidal, would have taken its toll on him.

The day my parents sat me down to tell me they were separating, the first thing I thought about was Nathan. Before I could feel anything about the devastation of their relationship, I was concerned with how it would affect my brother.

So even though there were tussles over the years between the two of us, there was always love.

After my work experience at the health retreat and before I'd taken the job back there, we went on our regular New Year's family holiday and Nathan and I had a huge fight. This was just after my 20th birthday and my brother was still adept at pushing my buttons. He said some things that made me snap and, in front of everyone, I really lost it. Instead of walking away, as I usually tried to do, I punched him hard in the arm and he jerked away with a loud cry. After that, we didn't speak a word to each other for three months. Not a word.

We returned to Sydney and then I headed off to my new job, not knowing how long I'd be gone. Nathan was turning 18 and about to embark on his final year of high school and the HSC. It would have been the occasion to bid a fond farewell to my brother, but he was having none of that.

Up at the retreat, I was pursuing a really healthy lifestyle and for the first few months I was focused on my purpose for being there. Everything was good until a couple of months in when I became sick. In this tropical paradise where I was eating well and being active, how could this be?

My mother hates it when we are ill, and she was fretting about my health. She'd been so used to having me under her wing and within her watch. Now I was away from home and I wasn't well, but she was powerless to intervene and help as she had so constantly been called to do over the past decade. And she'd had to be more vigilant than most mothers.

My nanna was also worried because she hated the fact that my brother and I weren't talking. Family harmony is paramount for her and family trumps

mum, i wish i was dead

everything. Our fighting was one of the worst things we could do to her. As her own brother and parents died when she was young, and she'd already lost her sister, she appreciates just how precious our family ties are. They shouldn't be jeopardised as carelessly as my brother and I were doing by our silence.

At the retreat, when I fell sick I knew that there was probably an emotional cause. It had been the case throughout my life. My constant battle with tonsillitis at school, the severe bouts of constipation and my inability to walk, these had all been manifestations of deeper emotional problems. I now know when I'm sick there's something not right in my life.

I spent about six weeks being really sick even though I was exercising and eating organic food. There was no reason why I should have been unwell physically because physically I was doing everything perfectly. So I knew my current poor health had an emotional basis. My health was declining and I didn't want to risk it getting any worse. I should have been on antibiotics, but that wasn't going to deal with the root problem. I had to figure out what that was.

When I was up at the retreat I'd learned how to meditate and switch my mind off completely, something I thought I'd never be able to do. I can turn it off and have a blank space without a single thought going through it.

I decided that I could solve this problem on my own without recourse to my psychologist back in Sydney. I thought: 'I have the tools to figure this out for myself. I just need time.'

So on one of my days off, I went to one of the empty rooms up there and I lay down and meditated for six hours, in two-hour blocks. I thought the problem was all leftover stuff from my previous relationship, the one that was really intense. I attempted to bring that to the surface and start thinking about it.

I was lying there, just thinking about my ex-girlfriend and the relationship, and then all of a sudden my brother came up. I was motionless for hours, just getting up for some food and water, then returning to my solitude.

As everything came to the foreground, tears were running down my cheeks. It was all about my brother, going back to when we were very young kids. I had always acknowledged what my parents had done and been through for me. My mother had been the main support and bore the brunt of coping with my depression. My dad had worked hard to provide financial security and the wherewithal for my care. I understood it logically and accepted everything they had both done. My nanna had been a day-to-day loving presence.

But I had never once stopped to realise what Nathan had done. I remember looking back and seeing him; his face was just fear and sadness, staring at me. Tears were in my eyes. I sifted through this stuff for hours, with all these flashbacks, remembering Nathan's involvement but only now seeing his role for what it was. How wrong I was about him. These tremendous feelings were coursing through me. It was the first time I acknowledged everything he went through and did for me. It was also the first time I acknowledged that I was jealous of him. It was a revelation.

Siblings don't admit they're jealous, they just pretend to be cool with each other. The next day I was much better; I was 100 per cent. I called mum and I told her all about it but I wasn't ready to speak with Nathan, so I wrote him a letter. I firmly believe that if you want to say something and get it off your chest, writing it out in a letter is a good way to formulate your thoughts. But do sleep on it first before sending, so that you can review what you've said when the heat is gone. I sent the letter to Nathan. His reply was brief: 'I read it'.

If I have something bothering me, I need to resolve it. I have to say and express what I need to. I can't ignore it; if I ignore it then it only gets worse or I get sick until I acknowledge the problem. This isn't about the response, if any, that I receive. What fixes things and allows me to move on is simply speaking my truth. Being honest with myself and accepting the situation is enough.

We never discussed it further. We didn't have to. Everything that had to be said had been said. He acknowledged the explanation for my behaviour and my apology for never having recognised his support and what I'd put him through. Ever since then, our relationship has been better than I'd ever believed it could possibly be.

At the time when we were growing up, I had all the attention from the age of 10 to 17. He was entering the turbulence of adolescence, going from 13 to 15 during the years of my intense depression and he still needed parenting. I had always sucked up 110 per cent of everyone's attention. Everyone wanted to know: 'Is Adam okay? Is Adam okay?' Nathan had nothing, and I never even considered that.

mum, i wish i was dead

We still have our arguments and fight. I think he can be lazy and selfish, and he thinks I overreact and care too much about things, but it's never been bad like that ever again.

It took a very long time to get there. That's what the serious sickness at the retreat was about, everything that was unresolved between my brother and me. Our relationship has been wonderful ever since. Before that reconciliation, our parents couldn't have left us alone together in the house when they went away. Afterwards, they took an overseas holiday for two months, and in that time we had only one argument. I feel very lucky to have such a good brother and to enjoy the relationship we have now.

We are both at university and, because of the years I was out of the education system, he's now ahead of me with his studies. He's in second year and I'm only in first. It's funny, for the first time in my life I'm asking my brother for advice. 'How do you do this reference ...?' He helps, he explains, punctuation and all that – he's very good and patient with me. We also speak about girls and he knows if he says something to me, I'm not going to tell our parents. I defend him as much as I can.

There is a sense of trust and love between us that I couldn't have imagined being possible several years ago. We both ask for each other's advice, whether it is about exercise, friends, university work, girls, or our parents. We may not always listen to the advice, but at least we can ask the questions. Although we may disagree on many issues, it only makes us stronger as it shows how far we have come. Where we used to scream and fight or not speak at all, we now have a mutually respectful and healthy relationship.

My letter to Nathan

So I'm not entirely sure how to be writing this, please read it all. Just so you know, I wanted to say all of what you're about to read, face to face. I just thought after everything that you would want to read this and absorb it all in your own time.

I don't know where exactly to start with this, but I'm just going to start somewhere. I'll probably repeat myself but it all needs to get out, and I realise how long over due this all is.

I want to say how sorry I am, for everything, for literally everything. It only all hit me the other week when I got extremely sick. I thought it was because of my ex and all the shit that happened when I got back the first time, and also just before I came up here again, but it wasn't. She was just a distraction from how I was feeling about you. I was meditating for about six hours, because for the first time I was up here, being sick made me stop and do what needed to be done.

I was lying there, breathing with nothing in particular on my mind. I tried to focus on what had happened with my ex but I never could focus; then out of the blue, you came into my mind, as did everything that had ever occurred between us. I literally mean everything!

The night on holidays recently, the time I flicked porridge on the wall and blamed you, the first time you asked me about girls, the time you called mum and dad in, 'crying' that I hurt you and I pulled the blanket off you and you had a massive smile on your face., every time I called you mushroom head, how proud I was of you watching you play soccer, running and coming first by a mile, every single time I screamed and got angry at you and seeing the look in your face of fear and sadness, the feeling I got sitting in hospital when mum and dad told me they were splitting up and the only thought going through my head was you being alone out there without me, playing basketball with you, going to *xxxx* (or however you spell it) and bike riding and catching fish, that time at *resort* on the Island with that stupid security guard and him touching you, followed by me smashing the bar, our first time to Bali after me having ECT, seeing you graduate primary school, the time I scared you so much you had to run up the street away from me, so many times you running away, the time you threw up everywhere, the times your friends threw up everywhere, Mardi Gras when I got the message from my ex at the time, and feeling so

mum, i wish i was dead

angry but so beyond worried at the same time, the time you scraped your chin at Coolum (or wherever the place was with the pools), the amounts of times while I was going through my depression how you kept out of my way and put up with all the horrible shit that I did and came out of my mouth and everything else, speaking to you while I was up here the first time just knowing you're ok and doing well made me feel so proud of everything you are doing, when you found out about your back and the disappointment that followed, over in France, all the skiing trips and the car ride down there in the land cruiser, all the games of pool and table tennis and the snow ball fights, the time when we used to go to the bagel shop at the corner when we lived in *xxxx*, the day before our house in *xxxx* got demolished and we went there with dad and threw rocks around, the time I came back from sleeping at my friend's house and found all my fish dead after you and *xxxx* overfed them, every time we wrestled, all the hours and hours of wrestling we used to watch, being at nanna's and building all the cubby houses out of all the furniture, the times we used to walk Windsor, the drive down to get Mindy, the time we went to Melbourne to watch the wrestling live, all the weekends at the 'family friends' learning how to swim followed by the roller blading, the hours of playing Mario cart and banjo kazooie with you, the street cricket, your barmitzvah and me going to Queensland getting the treatments with *xxxx* to attempt to be happy for that day …

I honestly remember everything. I could go on for pages and pages all the memories I had and the feelings that came with it, all the easy times and all the hard times, and there have been a fuckload of both, the best memory I have is of you, the very first time I saw you, in fact you are my very first memory.

I remember only being two and a half, the weather was overcast and lightly showering; dad and I went to this creepy toy store and bought you a green crocodile. We then went to the hospital to see mum, and there you were. That's the first memory I have, you.

Adam Schwartz   149

It all only hit me the other week just how much you have seen and been put through by me and everything I went through. I had always easily seen how much mum had done, even everything dad did and what they both went through. But naively, I had never even realised the effect everything had on you. Then it all hit me, everything that you had seen and done, you were 13 at the time! And for you to see me, your only brother wanting to die every day, on meds, gaining weight, changed personality, angry, aggressive, sad, the list goes on and on and I'm sure your remember it all – it must have been indescribable.

It hit me: every time I have ever yelled at you, made you so afraid you cried, run away or hid from me. I went straight back to that moment and for the first time I saw it from your perspective, and took the look you had on your face. I felt what you felt and I burst out into tears, realising everything I had done and how I had made you feel.

What I went through was something that no one had any control over, and I'm not apologising for what I went through. I'm apologising for how it affected your life to this very point in time. What I had I had for years before it got as bad as it was. And you probably have never known this: growing up, I was beyond jealous of you in every way.

You could eat anything you wanted and not gain a single gram, you have always been naturally amazing at sport, you always had dad's love and a much better relationship with him, had always been popular, confident and always great with girls, the family friends loved you, had lots of friends – from my view you had everything and simply flew through life without a care.

None of this was your fault, you have never done anything wrong, but from my view at that age, I had this huge jealousy, which I didn't understand. I had this hatred for you because I felt like such an outcast, and no matter how hard I tried I never was great at sport, every food that went into my mouth turned into fat, every girl I liked never liked me back. I was constantly comparing myself to you and

mum, i wish i was dead

was so jealous and angry. You never did a single thing wrong, you were simply being you and there's nothing wrong with that. You have always been an amazing kid; you achieve everything you set out to do, you fly through things I have always found beyond hard. After growing up from that my jealousy turned to being simply just proud of you.

Those two years, at the height of my depression, all those feelings had been made 100 times worse. I felt hatred towards you simply because I hated myself, and that you had always found life so easy and yet here I was suffering every day. What I had never realised until recently is that everything I went through happened for a reason and if I could, I wouldn't change a thing because of everything I have learned and have gained form that experience. The only problem had been that I never stopped and appreciated you, everything that my depression made you go through, everything that I used to put onto you, everything that you used to see, hear and experience – all the attention that was taken away from you because I needed so much damn care at the time.

Mum and dad, the family friends, no adults truly understood what was happening, let alone a 13-year-old kid. It must have been horrible and I can only imagine how hard it was. I put myself in your shoes and how I would have felt seeing you suffer and want to die every day. You losing your friends, seeing you get so angry for no reason, seeing my only brother scream down my throat for no reason at all, the never knowing when a good moment was, simply imagining you in hospital alone and feeling everything I remember feeling, all the judgement from friends, me feeling I have to run away from my own home to feel safe, not knowing what to do because every action seemed to make you angry … just thinking and imagining all that, I couldn't stop crying. I have had years of counselling following the ECT to help me get over and understand everything that happened. You haven't had anything. It all has just been bottled up.

I realised, being up north, that life will keep presenting lessons and those lessons will repeat until what's needed to be learned is learned. Odd moments over the recent few years I have snapped at you, giving me the chance to stop, learn and realise what I'm doing all over again, but I never had until now.

There is no excuse for anything and I can't change the past. And even if I could, I wouldn't because I genuinely believe that no matter how hard life gets and how unfair it seems, that everything is happening for reasons we can never truly understand until the lesson has been learned and enough time has passed to look back on a situation and understand it. Everything that has ever happened to me has led me to this point and I wouldn't change a thing.

I need you to know how sorry I am for everything. You are a typical teenage kid, you are living that life, going to parties, drinking everything kids at your age should be doing, I was put through a very different path. I remember getting so angry on Mardi Gras and all those other times involving you going out and being a normal teenager because you are my brother, and all those other kids doing that stuff I see as stupid kids. But in my eyes you're not stupid, you're smart and your potential is limitless! However, I was stupid in thinking that what you were doing was wrong. It wasn't and never has been; you are just experiencing a different path to me and learning what you need to learn in your own ways and in your own time. I was naively holding you to this standard and expectations I held for myself, and that was really wrong.

My depression made my emotions all over the place, and I would react on such an extreme level to everything and everyone. If I liked someone it was all of a sudden love, if something annoyed me I then hated that person, I was so paranoid, so self-conscious, so fucked up that I wouldn't even want you to begin to understand how internally messed up I was. So whenever you would do normal things that typical brothers would do, I would react and snap in ways that most brothers would never do.

　　　　　　　　　　　　　　　mum, i wish i was dead

I truly am sorry for all the pain I have caused you, for every tear you have ever shed because of my actions, every time you felt so scared you had to run away, every time you had to explain my actions to a friend, every time you had to lie because of me.

Sorry for not stopping and appreciating how my life has so drastically affected yours.

I'm beyond sorry for not realising how much you have done for me my entire life, giving me space when I needed, leaving when I needed, not fighting back, growing up in a home with someone who wasn't emotionally stable. The list just goes on and on and on of everything you have done, the smiles you gave me, the encouragement, the inspiration. Much like mum and nanna, you were one of the only three reasons I held onto my life, that I didn't jump off the balcony or push myself down the stairs, or walk in front of a bus. Having you in my life truly saved my life.

I love you like words can't describe. Not speaking to you, not knowing how you are, not having you come to me for advice left a hole in me I didn't know could exist.

I'm so sorry for so much, for the pain I have caused you, the trauma you experienced, the suffering you saw me go through, the abuse you took, not realising and appreciating what you went through and the endless things you have done for me and given me.

I have probably repeated myself and unfortunately missed out on a lot of things, and I'm sure reading this won't have nearly as much truth to it as if you could see me saying this to you, seeing how much emotion this brings up in me as I write all this.

You are a normal kid and I was the abnormal one. I couldn't stop or change what I went through, and I know that's not my fault, but I know how much it affected you. It isn't my fault what I went through, and at the same time it's not your fault for you being who you are. What I went through made me react in ways normal people, normal brothers, would never have reacted. Just because I had no control over what was happening to me and everything was so extreme that I didn't understand, still doesn't make it right or fair that you had to be witness and a part of that and be on the receiving end of my anger, sadness and all those emotions that would come out.

You are my only brother, you are my family, you will be the uncle to my kids and I'll be the uncle to yours, you will always be in my life and that won't change, I just want us to be happy with each other, be able to laugh and joke around, to be able to speak to each other on a deeper level when needed, to come to each other for advice, to move on from everything that has happened. I understand that it's easier said than done, but I hope this is the first step to at least trying.

I'm not expecting anything back from you; I just wanted you to know all of that and how truly beyond sorry I am. These words don't even come close to saying how deeply I feel and simply that I love you unconditionally. No matter what trouble you ever get into, whatever drugs you end up taking, amounts of alcohol you drink, who you date, what you say, where you end up and whatever path you end up leading, I will always be there for you and I will always love you.

20

My Life from Now

The world of physical fitness had paved a road out of my old life into the new. Through exercise and psychology sessions, I had returned to physical and emotional good health. It was also the environment in which I was able to forge a closer relationship with my father and, more recently, my brother. It's easy for two men to head off to the gym together. It gives purpose to socialising and allows you to talk while you are on a treadmill or lifting weights.

Strange that these activities should have been part of my salvation when it was in the realm of sport, albeit competitive, that I endured so much frustration and disappointment as I was growing up.

More than this, exercise has provided me with employment as a trainer, so I was able to earn an income and pay my way. I left school without any qualifications and no idea where I could go, and very quickly was filling my hours in work that I genuinely enjoyed. I felt very lucky.

While I can't see a time when I won't be seriously committed to an exercise regime, at the age of 20 I realised I wanted to seek a profession in which I could use my head. I didn't want to search for another job so again I consulted with a careers adviser. The one who had introduced me to personal training was not available, so I met up with another this time, a man.

Behind the scenes, my mother had been doing a lot of research on what was out there for me. This is her method of smoothing the way for me. She does all the legwork and then presents all the information for me. So even before I'd set foot in the careers adviser's office, she'd scanned the scene. One thing she'd discovered is that if I wanted to go on to study at university, a number of places require you to have sat the STAT – the Standard Tertiary Admission Test.

It's a test that you can't really study for and is primarily focused on IQ. My mum's view was that I should explore what was available and keep my options open, and since the STAT was an essential prerequisite for some of those options, it was best to get it done and out of the way. Then it was there if needed, once I'd decided what I wanted to study.

The careers adviser recommended several of the big universities in Sydney, as well as one up in Queensland. I did think about the Queensland university because I still have a lot of friends up there from my time at the health retreat, but I knew that I would really need the support of my family to get me through the potential challenges I would face. In the end, a university on Sydney's north shore was the way I went; it was a less conservative and more flexible institution compared with the heritage sandstone universities.

Without my Higher School Certificate, I chose to enrol through the non-award route, which meant a half-load for a year as a mature age student. If I did well, I could then take on a full load in my second year. Success in the STAT would help get me straight in with a full load. That's the way I went.

I felt very nervous the night before sitting the STAT. I hadn't done an exam for four years and this was a serious one with my entrance to uni riding on it. I felt so nervous the night before and on the day. Once over, it was nerve-wracking waiting for the results.

A friend who was already studying at my new uni took me for a look around. The feel of the place, a more sprawling green campus than its inner city counterparts, was very welcoming.

Mature-age students could enter this university through the Jubilee program via Bachelor of Arts, Bachelor of Science or Bachelor of Teaching (Early Childhood Education) programs. I chose to enrol in a Bachelor of Arts as you can do anything in arts; you don't need to pick your major straightaway. I would be able to taste and see what I liked. This got me excited because I wouldn't have to do something I found boring. From my past experience, I knew that if a course didn't stimulate me, I would be disinclined to keep up with my studies.

When I attended the uni open day, a student adviser ran through a list of possible courses, with everything from science to business. I excitedly looked up course codes and abstracts, hungry for the choices on offer.

In the first semester I decided to do a bit of everything. I had no idea what I would like or want to learn about, so I chose a variety of topics that looked tempting. My schedule included philosophy, media, brain science, and academic learning in the humanities. The last of these taught you how to write essays – a skill which I had yet to master. It was a subject you got points for so I thought I should do it because it was going to teach me everything I needed to know for uni.

After that semester I realised I really loved philosophy and enjoyed studying it. I was still the kid who had turned up to Michelle's garage for her art class who wanted to talk about the meaning of life. So in my second semester, I did both of the only two philosophy subjects available, as well as sociology and marketing. And I loved the philosophy. It's going to give me the motivation to keep going to uni. I wouldn't stay if I were doing something I found painstaking. I couldn't put the effort in.

The first semester was painful and my head would physically hurt. I was drained. I couldn't do anything else but fulfil my study requirements. I hadn't used my brain to learn anything in that way for a very, very long time. Sitting exams didn't cause me any worry, though I am still anxious while awaiting my results. Tutors would tell me how good I was at expressing myself when I was talking, but I would lose a lot of quality when I put my thoughts on paper. That upset me. Writing an essay didn't show how well I could communicate verbally. My essay writing improved dramatically over the year but it still wasn't good enough.

Uni proved a challenge because it brought up a lot of unresolved issues that I hadn't realised I was still clinging onto. Principal among these was the sense of failure I had felt when I left school, believing I had let go of my education. I had thought that the only way to get into uni and be successful in life was completing high school and getting the HSC. At the time, I'd rationalised that I really didn't have a choice about staying on because with my memory loss I was incapable of study, but it was a real blow to my self-esteem. I'd had to limit my horizons and think in terms of getting through the next few months, instead of focusing on a bright future.

It was reassuring to get through my first year at uni and it was good to be that little bit older than my fellow students. I wanted to do well and a pass wasn't going to be good enough for me.

Some of the things that frustrated me in the real world were also represented in the microcosm of the uni, such as having a tutor you don't like. Because you are beholden to them as the person who has the power to grade you, it is the same as having a manager at work whom you don't see eye to eye with. Although I've developed some skills around these relationships, it is still very frustrating when you want to communicate your opinion and speak out.

Being older, I have learned to let go. You ask a question and if you are wrong, you learn from it. So I am always happy to ask questions in tutorials and run the risk of looking foolish while the kids straight out of high school are too scared to ask. They'll just sit there in silence for an hour. Having that experience in the outside world benefited me and I had an advantage.

mum, i wish i was dead

21

The Importance of Awareness

The most important message I can pass on to anyone reading this is: awareness. Not just self-awareness, but general awareness of others and your environment. To understand not only how you work, but also what works best for you. It is the foundation that has allowed me to maintain my health to this day. It is impossible for any one person to have all the answers for every other person. In fact, the only person who can really have all the answers for yourself is you.

Self-awareness and its necessity is something I had to learn relatively early on. The consequence of dealing with a mental illness is not having an objective scan or blood test that can determine exactly what it was and how to treat it. Once I realised this, and after a few sessions with my psychiatrist, it became clear that my diagnosis and treatment was heavily reliant on how I could describe how I was feeling. The more aware I was of myself, how I was feeling and what I reacted to, the better I could describe how I was internally to my doctor. With this came the development and understanding of words associated with my emotions so the description I was giving was as accurate as it could be. The better my description, then the more accurate the diagnosis, which led to more appropriate and (hopefully) effective treatment.

My self-awareness didn't develop by choice; it was a necessity for survival and has helped me in all areas of my life to this day. It has both allowed and forced me to learn a variety of tools and techniques to maintain my health and overall wellbeing. Yes, some may work for you too, but many may not. Everyone is unique; we may have similar experiences but we will always be different. That means what works for me may be different to what works for you and vice versa. You can't learn a life lesson unless you live it.

And that's okay! Despite our desire to want to 'fit in' and to be accepted by our peers and communities, we will always have our differences. It is important to remember and embrace that there is only one of you, much like there is only one of me. No one will ever be as good at being me than me, much like there is no one out there who can be as good at being you, than you. We are each truly unique. Our uniqueness should be loved and celebrated, not hidden due to shame or embarrassment.

There are several general foundations to be aware of. Have good, clear communication with those around and supporting you. Be physically active and have regular exercise. Have an eating pattern that consists of nutritious food. Make sure sleep is consistent and regular. It may seem obvious to some that having good sleep, regular exercise, healthy diet and good communication skills is an easy, general regime that anyone could follow and live a 'good' life. However, this should be used as a guideline. What is most important is for an individual to figure out how and what works best for them.

The tools I have learned made a significant difference both in my recovery and my life generally. Not just when I was suffering intensely with depression but the years following, up until this point. This has allowed me to consistently maintain my health and live a life free from the restrictions depression once imposed on me.

When I was really bad, one of the main areas we (my mother and I) had to improve on was communication – how she communicated with me and how I communicated with her. Not that my mum had anything wrong with her communication skills with most people. I just wasn't most people. I was severely depressed, with irrational, chaotic thoughts. Usual communication was not working for me, as during these periods I received and interpreted things quite differently. She had to learn new ways of effectively communicating with me.

I continuously found myself in a position of conflict (more so than usual). I had originally promised my mum that if anything ever got really bad, as in I wanted to die, that I must always tell her so I can get the help I need. Although I kept my promise, it was getting harder and harder to keep. I never wanted to hurt anyone, I was suffering and I could see, if not sense, what that suffering was doing to the people I loved. I didn't want to make it worse for them.

Every time I wanted to die, felt horrific, needed to get my morbid, angry, hopeless thoughts out of my head, I kept my promise and told her. However, despite my mum's best efforts I could always see how much it pained her knowing how bad I actually was. This made me feel even worse. I never wanted to hurt anyone, especially my mother.

I believe it was the psychologist she was seeing at the time who provided her with support, which initially suggested emails as an effective tool in communication. This arose because any time mum had to tell me anything, even something as simple as notifying me of an appointment, or positive encouragement, it would anger me. Due to the depression I couldn't handle any forms of requests or suggestions. I received it all irrationally, as accusations, and the pressure I felt would cause me stress above and beyond what I was already feeling.

These two reasons led to the best thing regarding our communication that could have happened. People complain how emotionless technology has made communication (email, text messaging, and so on). However, this same reason made it the perfect tool. Emailing took away the intensity of what face-to-face conversations brought up. It allowed mum to share with me important information that I would be able to read and receive in my own time when I was calm, and if needed, respond. Most importantly from my perspective, it allowed me to keep my promise. I always felt I could be open and share anything I was feeling with mum. It stopped me from having to see that distraught look my mum had when I shared my morbid feelings with her. It allowed our communication to stay open.

Moving on after the intense depression and ECT treatment, the combination of my perfectionist personality, as well as fear of and the desire to do everything possible to prevent a severe depressive episode again, I had to learn and accept not just what I went through, but who I am as a person. Change the things I could and wanted to, as well as love the things I couldn't and didn't want to change.

Initially I would get very concerned anytime I felt bad. Even just a slight dip in my mood would have me worrying that it would turn into a depression.

Every time I got angry, sad, annoyed or sick, the same concern would arise. First, I had to learn that feeling these emotions meant I was human and *not* becoming depressed and that these emotions are 'normal'. Concern would arise when these feelings compounded for several days in a row. When this happened, instead of getting worried like I previously had, I learned how to look at the bigger picture – my life as a whole, not one or two possible factors. I learned to accept the darkness and not be fearful or fight the feelings that come with it. Trying to suppress and deny it only made everything worse for me and all it did was extend the depressive episode. Once I stop and acknowledge what is happening, I can then face it and resolve it, allowing me to move forward.

I learned what an impact the weather has on my mood. The difference between what I am like in summer and winter used to be like two different people. I realise how much of a positive influence the sun, as well as the beach, has on my mood. So now I put things in place during winter to maintain my mood, as well as be aware of possible emotional dips. This includes the food I eat, my physical activity, having things to look forward to and appointments with my psychologist if needed.

Now I know the effect certain foods have on me, especially sugar. When consumed on a regular basis, sugar not only affects my sleep, weight gain and skin, it has a negative effect on my mood. I become more irritable and lazy, long term. On that same note, exercise has had a huge impact on my life. Beyond the weight loss, physical health and vanity, when it is done regularly, my mood is always better. I am more relaxed, happier, more energised and focused, positive and have better sleep patterns. Lack of exercise seemingly has the opposite effect. I become aggressive, lazy, tired, distracted, unfocused and find it hard to maintain good sleep.

Sleep – regular, deep sleep – is vital. Several days without proper sleep affects not just my mood but energy levels, food cravings and irritability.

It's imperative to understand how important relationships affect me, both friendship and romantically. If things go bad – a break-up, a fight, a disagreement – I needed to learn how to manage myself and the intense emotions that could arise. Much like in winter, I have tools in place to help.

One thing I was always fearful of was that I would never be 'normal' – normal in the sense of being able to fit in. I already felt like such an outsider after the depression, ECT and not finishing high school. I was afraid that I wouldn't be able to 'fit in' socially. At the ages of 17 and 18, the biggest thing socially is partying, going out and having some drinks with friends.

I was always warned about hard drugs, cocaine, pills, etc. They could very easily alter my mood, especially because my depression was a chemical imbalance, the down from coming off any of them could trigger a snowball effect into another depressive episode. No high would ever be worth even the slightest chance of dipping again. I have an unwavering desire to not dip again, especially after all the hard work I put in already to maintain my health. This kept me from ever even considering doing those drugs. So I never did. Although I was warned about alcohol, it was to be careful, rather than to avoid. Also to be aware that different alcohol affects people differently.

The last point I learned from people's comments of how I was when I went out, what I remembered and how I felt the following day, not hangover-wise, but emotionally. I learned that certain alcohol has no negative emotional effects on me at all. On that same note, I learned that there are several alcohols that have a dire effect on my mood. So I could still go out and be 'normal' and seemingly 'fit in'. I drank the drinks that had no effect, and the ones that made everything worse, I simply avoided.

I was always raised with 'if you don't have something nice to say, then don't say it at all'. A noble sentiment that may be, but it is not the rule people conduct themselves by. I learned very quickly that I cannot control people around me, their actions, what they say, or their intent behind it all. People are going to say what they want to say and do what they want to do. They will tease, bully, be backhanded, lie, cheat, aggravate, get upset, annoy others or feel anger – the list goes on. The only thing I had any control over was *me*. Yet I found myself reacting to other people's opinions about me.

I had made a promise to myself to never let anyone make me feel as bad as I had let myself feel. Yet, here I was, reacting to people, to their negativity towards me, as well as feeling this need to have people's approval. I didn't have control of it. I would just feel whatever it was in that situation. I couldn't blame them even if they had bad intentions. I was reacting and I didn't know why.

The promise I made to myself drove me to resolve these issues. In every situation I felt unnecessarily negative about myself I would remember it, see my psychologist and resolve it. The techniques he used meant the issue that originally brought up the problem never arose again. Even to this day when something arises that I can't resolve on my own, I use the same process to resolve it.

Realising that opinion is not fact was a huge revelation. Even experts in their field regularly have differing opinions. Yet at one stage of my life I was taking people's opinions about me to be fact –people who had zero expertise in any field. People I didn't even know, could hurt me with words I gave value to. As soon as I removed the value of their opinion, I retook control of what I let affect me.

Ironically, in a weird way, I look forward to feeling 'off', if only because it gives me a chance to learn something new about myself. The greatest things I have been able to do for myself haven't come from other people but have come from persistence in figuring out who I am and what works best for me. The lessons I've learned have come from me. I definitely needed help reaching each place of understanding, but it has been a crucial role in being as emotionally healthy as I am today.

I don't have all the answers; I'm still learning myself. It is impossible to have all the answers to get through depression, to lead a healthy life. There is no magic pill or realisation that fixes everything. It is hard, very hard. It's an invisible battle that affects more people than is realised. It can end lives. It can destroy families. True understanding can only come from experiencing its depths. Ask anyone who has suffered and they wouldn't wish it upon their worst enemy. Despite all this, there is hope. It takes work but it is possible.

Nevertheless, I wouldn't change a thing, even if I could. I would choose to suffer each day again because it has led me to this point. It has taught me invaluable lessons, not just about myself and who I am, but about life as well. It brought my family closer together, to a point I never thought possible. I have met some amazing people and shared many stories. It has allowed me to help others going through similar situations. I have been able to write this book, intending to help many more.

I love myself and accept who I am. I cannot change the past nor would I want to. We all have a journey and lessons to learn along the way. My experiences have been unique, yet my struggle is all too common. I accept it as a part of me, but I refuse to let it define me.

22

Back to the Beginning

I've been on an incredible and painful journey. Although it has been difficult and long, I've ended up exactly where I started from. Nothing has changed, and yet everything feels different.

I still live in the same house I grew up in and which I once despised. I fall asleep every night in the bedroom whose walls and furnishings I used to attack. The room has withstood the repeated destructive onslaughts over those terrible years with little evidence to show for it. The scars have been repaired. The room I cried myself to sleep in on too many nights, the room I was fearful of waking up in, is the same room I now fall quietly to sleep in.

In summer, I sit on the balcony enjoying the sunshine; the very same balcony I imagined throwing myself from. Every day I walk up and down the stairs where I used to see myself lying dead at the bottom of. The streets I walk around the neighbourhood are still as busy with cars but I no longer want to jump in front of them. The drivers pass me by harmlessly as they go about their way and I go about mine. Our lives won't be inextricably linked through some horrible suicide 'deal' in which they become an unwitting player.

I still see the people who knew me at my lowest point. Now when we socialise it's to share a laugh and enjoy each other's company. The dinner table I sit at with friends and family is the same one I slammed my fists on before storming from the house and spiralling into the abyss. Only now we are sharing a joke and talking excitedly about our plans for the weekend and our busy lives.

Today, I look in the same mirror and smile at the reflection that used to make me cry.

So many people run away and think things will get better if they replace old surroundings with new. You can run away from a bad situation, but when the problem lies within yourself, wherever you go the problem goes with you.

Here's the thing: the world around me is more or less the same. It's me who has changed. I have managed this disease out of existence.

I am still here, yet my world and how I experience it has changed entirely. I know I can't undo the past. I don't want to. It's a part of who I am. But slowly, day-by-day, I am creating a new life, and with it a bank of happy memories. I am now excited and hopeful for my future and the new challenges that lie ahead. A future I never thought possible.

For more information, go to **www.adamschwartz.com.au**

mum, i wish i was dead

Lightning Source UK Ltd.
Milton Keynes UK
UKOW06f1620190615

253798UK00013B/184/P